COVID-19

Peter Murphy

COVID-19

Proportionality, Public Policy and Social Distancing

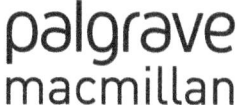

Peter Murphy
La Trobe University
Bundorra, VIC, Australia

ISBN 978-981-15-7516-7   ISBN 978-981-15-7514-3 (eBook)
https://doi.org/10.1007/978-981-15-7514-3

© The Editor(s) (if applicable) and The Author(s), under exclusive licence to Springer Nature Singapore Pte Ltd. 2020
This work is subject to copyright. All rights are solely and exclusively licensed by the Publisher, whether the whole or part of the material is concerned, specifically the rights of translation, reprinting, reuse of illustrations, recitation, broadcasting, reproduction on microfilms or in any other physical way, and transmission or information storage and retrieval, electronic adaptation, computer software, or by similar or dissimilar methodology now known or hereafter developed.
The use of general descriptive names, registered names, trademarks, service marks, etc. in this publication does not imply, even in the absence of a specific statement, that such names are exempt from the relevant protective laws and regulations and therefore free for general use.
The publisher, the authors and the editors are safe to assume that the advice and information in this book are believed to be true and accurate at the date of publication. Neither the publisher nor the authors or the editors give a warranty, expressed or implied, with respect to the material contained herein or for any errors or omissions that may have been made. The publisher remains neutral with regard to jurisdictional claims in published maps and institutional affiliations.

Cover pattern © Melissa Hasan

This Palgrave Pivot imprint is published by the registered company Springer Nature Singapore Pte Ltd.
The registered company address is: 152 Beach Road, #21-01/04 Gateway East, Singapore 189721, Singapore

ACKNOWLEDGEMENT

I wrote a preliminary report on COVID-19 in April 2020 for *Budhi: A Journal of Ideas and Culture*. Material from that article is used here with kind permission.

CONTENTS

1	Social Distance	1
2	Public Policy	39
3	Social Mood	85
	Afterword	107
	Index	117

ABOUT THE AUTHOR

Peter Murphy is the author of *The Political Economy of Prosperity*, *Limited Government*, *Auto-Industrialism*, *Universities and Innovation Economies*, and *The Collective Imagination*, among other books. He is Adjunct Professor of Humanities and Social Sciences, La Trobe University, Australia, and Adjunct Professor in The Cairns Institute at James Cook University. He writes on public policy and social theory.

List of Tables

Table 1.1	Nursing home deaths as a percentage of total COVID-related deaths	5
Table 1.2	European mortality, excess deaths, z-scores, March–April 2020	8
Table 1.3	COVID-19, selected countries, deaths per million population and contextual factors, May 27, 2020	9
Table 1.4	COVID-19 infection fatality rates (IFR) and projected resulting deaths among infected national populations	13
Table 1.5	COVID-19 conjectured contextual factors: which, if any, factors correlate with country deaths per million?	16
Table 1.6	Air pollution by major COVID-19 affected cities, 2016	18
Table 1.7	Air passengers by major COVID-19 affected cities, 2018	18
Table 1.8	Preferred interpersonal social distancing and COVID-19, selected countries	23
Table 1.9	Europe, comparative locations, preferred interpersonal social distancing, 2014, centimetres	25
Table 1.10	High-contact culture: US and Canada	26
Table 1.11	Italy COVID-19 deaths per capita by region May 26, 2020 compared with population density and civic intensity	30
Table 2.1	Number of COVID-19 tests per million by country and date	40
Table 2.2	Early COVID-19 mitigation actions taken December–March 2020	42
Table 2.3	Workplace location visits and length of stay against a baseline of Jan 3–Feb 6, 2020 activity	44
Table 2.4	Retail and recreation location visits and length of stay against a baseline of Jan 3–Feb 6, 2020 activity	45
Table 2.5	Germany, effective reproduction number of COVID-19 compared with government actions taken	51

Table 2.6	COVID-19 infection peak compared to lockdown timing	52
Table 2.7	Early models of the COVID-19 infection fatality rate (IFR) and projected resulting deaths assuming 60% of the population is infected	53
Table 2.8	Australia, ICU and ward beds for COVID-19 peak, predicted and actual	55
Table 2.9	IHME projected mean hospital COVID-19 beds needed vs actual COVID-19 serious and critical care hospitalisations, United States	56
Table 2.10	Comparison of the projected loss of life-span years from COVID-19 deaths [Imperial College model] with the loss of life-span years from unemployment in a major recession, United Kingdom	57
Table 2.11	IHME projected mean cumulative COVID-19 deaths vs actual COVID-19 deaths, United States	59
Table 2.12	Purchasing Managers Index (PMI), manufacturing by country, expansion and contraction	70
Table 2.13	Purchasing Managers Index (PMI), services by country, expansion and contraction	71
Table 2.14	Near-term visible expressions of long-term pathways to deaths of despair	74

CHAPTER 1

Social Distance

Abstract The chapter reviews primary-source virological and epidemiological studies to profile the COVID-19 virus. Key epidemiological concepts are introduced and various methods of mitigating viruses are discussed. The social nature of virus communicability and the roles of interpersonal distance and high-contact cultures as media for the transmission of the virus are detailed.

Keywords Social distance • High-contact culture • Clusters • Immunity • Crowds • Reproduction number • Family • Home • Death • Mortality • Nursing homes • Pathogen • Proxemics • High-touch societies • Social connections • Strangers • Transmission

1.1 2020

2020 will be remembered by contemporaries like 1989, 2001 and 2008 were. These were years of exogenous shocks. Societies and economies were roiled by big external events. In 1989 it was the collapse of the Soviet Union. In 2001, terrorism. In 2008, the sub-prime mortgage crisis. Each event triggered a fallout that cast a long shadow over the succeeding decade. All manner of dislocations, reconfigurations, adjustments and adaptations followed as societies scrambled to cope with a big jolt and make sense of it. In 2020 a similar exogenous shock was provided by the

© The Author(s) 2020
P. Murphy, *COVID-19*,
https://doi.org/10.1007/978-981-15-7514-3_1

COVID-19 (SARS-CoV-2) virus.[1] It set off a cascading series of interventions, restrictions and disruptions that culminated in the lockdown of whole societies and economies. What happened, why did it happen and was it justified? To answer these questions, we must begin with the virus itself.

1.2 Mortality

The degree of virulence of a virus can be measured. The standard measure—the R_0 [R-zero] or basic reproduction number of a virus—is the average number of persons that an average infected person can *potentially* infect. The effective reproduction number (R_E) tells us how many persons an average infected person *actually* infects at a given point (or points) in time.[2] The R_0 number assumes that there are otherwise no measures or conditions that limit the virus' communicability. The profile of the susceptible population, the behaviour of transmitting agents, and degrees of immunity can all affect the rate of spread of a virus in practice. An R_0 below 1 means that an infected person infects on average less than one person—and when that happens the virus struggles to reproduce itself and spread.

The basic reproduction number varies depending on the virus. The R_0 of mumps is high (4–12) though not as high as measles (12–18) or chicken pox (10–12). The 2019 H1N1 influenza R_0 was 1.4. Seasonal influenza ranges from 0.9 to 2.1 (Eisenberg 2020, February 5). The early estimates of the R_0 of COVID-19 varied widely. Oxford University's Centre for Evidence Based Medicine on April 14 2020 cited a median figure of 2.63 and an R_0 ranging from 0.4 to 4.6 (Aronson et al. 2020). This was based on nine early studies from Wuhan, Shenzhen and South Korea. In comparison, the 1918 pandemic flu had an R_0 of 2 to 3.

By assuming a given R_0 number, epidemiologists can derive from that a presumptive figure for the level of immunity that is potentially needed across society before a virus is unable to effectively reproduce itself. Infected persons if they don't die acquire immunity to re-infection. The susceptible population at a certain point begins to decline—and the virus increasingly struggles to reproduce itself. This is community immunity—or herd immunity. If the R_0 figure for COVID-19 was 2.63 then it was calculable that 62% of that population would need (in one way or another) to be immune in order for COVID-19 to die out (Aronson et al. 2020). That presupposed that no other factor reduced the person-to-person communicability of the virus.

The level of community immunity varies from virus to virus. In the case of mumps, given its high R_0 number, 75–86% of a population potentially needs to have immunity, either by virtue of a vaccine or the body's own antibodies, for the reproduction of the virus to fall low enough (below an R_0 of 1) for the transmission of the virus to slow and eventually stop. The R_0 figure has limits. It indicates the potential virulence of a virus. But this potential exists in the absence informal social adaptation, government control measures or environmental (e.g. hygiene, ventilation) factors that work to reduce the R_0 to an R_E—the latter being a measure of the virus' actual rather than just potential capacity to transmit from one person to one or more other persons. Models of R_0 that extrapolate from periods and places of uninhibited (maximum) spread of a virus do not necessarily reflect the communicability of the virus over its entire infectious history.

Immunity to a virus is achieved in several ways. The first is pharmaceutical: a vaccine against the virus. The second is exposure. Individuals who have not been vaccinated (or those for whom a vaccine is ineffective) are exposed to the virus. They then get sick and their own immune system responds. If their immune system successfully fights off the virus, they recover. The "memory" of their successful immune response is stored in their body in the form of B cell and IgA anti-bodies and memory T cells. Should the recovered person get exposed to the virus again, antibodies immediately tell their immune system what to do in order to repel the virus. T cells organize bodily immune defences and attacks. Vaccines take molecules (antigens) from the pathogen and introduce them into the body. This teaches the immune system to produce antibodies that will "remember" the viral pathogen in the future and act swiftly to repel it before the pathogen spreads and causes an illness.

When a person is exposed to a virus, one of four things happens: (a) they fall ill—in a small percentage of cases seriously or critically ill—and in a very small percentage of cases they will die; (b) they get exposed, have mild symptoms and recover; (c) they are asymptotic and never know that they were exposed and carried the virus;[3] (d) they have a vaccine shot, and the vaccine trains their immune system to successfully fight off the virus. Vaccines are often ineffective among aged populations over 70 with compromised immune systems.

Just as immunity to a virus varies across a population, so does susceptibility. Which part of a population is more susceptible or less susceptible to a virus also varies between different viruses. In the case of COVID-19-related deaths, these were concentrated among persons over 70 years of age (and especially among those over 80) who had multiple co-morbidities (underlying chronic conditions, notably high blood pressure, cardiovascular disease and diabetes).[4] In the United Kingdom for example, as of June 9 2020, 27,706 patients had died in hospital in England and tested positive for COVID-19. Of those persons, 95% had comorbidities, 53% were over 80 years old and 38% were aged between 60 and 79.[5]

This susceptibility profile was compounded—or reinforced—by social factors. Variously high and very high percentages of national and regional deaths from COVID-19 occurred in nursing homes (Table 1.1). A study of one American (Seattle) residential aged nursing home found that COVID-19 spread rapidly through the facility. Twenty-three days after the first positive test result for the COVID virus in the facility, 57 of the 89 residents (64%) tested positive (Arons et al. 2020, April 24). As of April 26 2020, in the countries where there was available official data on nursing homes—Australia, Belgium, Canada, France, Hungary, Ireland, Israel, Norway, Portugal, Singapore and some regions of Spain—the percentage of COVID-related deaths in care homes ranged from 19% to 72% (Comas-Herrera et al. 2020, April 26). As of late April 2020 in the United States 64% of Colorado's COVID-related deaths were in nursing homes and more than 50% in Connecticut (Wingerter 2020, April 22; Phaneuf 2020, April 20). The Foundation for Research on Equal Opportunity tabulated all nursing home/residential care deaths from COVID reported through to May 20 2020 in the United States. The Foundation calculated that 53.6% of all these deaths were in nursing homes (the figure excluded New York State as that state counted as hospital deaths nursing home residents who died in hospital) (Girvan and Roy 2020, May 8 & 22).[6] Nursing home residents make up 0.5% of the US population but over half of the COVID-related deaths in the United States (Table 1.1). As with all things COVID, the level of nursing home mortality that was associated with the virus ranged widely—from 81% of total deaths in Minnesota and 75% in Rhode Island to 35% in Tennessee and 32% in South Carolina. A comparable range applied internationally—from 11% in Singapore and 25% in Australia to 62% in Ireland and 82% in Canada (Table 1.1).

Principally old and especially very old persons had a high risk of dying if they were infected with the COVID-19 virus. That however raised the question of causality. For while many persons might die *with* the virus recorded on their death certificate, it remained an open question whether they necessarily died *because of* the virus. It was possible—and perhaps likely—that anywhere between a half and two-thirds of those in the high-risk cohort (i.e. aged persons with multiple underlying conditions) who

Table 1.1 Nursing home deaths as a percentage of total COVID-related deaths

Nation	COVID-19 death rate per million population, May 27 2020	Deaths in nursing homes as a % of total COVID-related deaths, May 22 2020	Long term residential care beds per million persons	Long term residential care beds as a % of total population	US State	COVID-19 death rate per million population, May 27 2020	Deaths in nursing homes as a % of total COVID-related deaths, May 12 2020
United Kingdom	546	55%a	8028	0.8%	New Jersey	1261	52.8%
France	437	50.9%	10,004	1.0%	Connecticut	1057	58.7%
Swedenb	408	48.9%	12,539	1.3%	Massachusetts	939	61.9%
United States	304	53.6%c	4966	0.5%	Louisiana	581	39.4%
Canada	176	82.1%	9033	0.9%	Pennsylvania	406	69.2%
Germany	101	37.4%	11,367	1.1%	Illinois	388	50.1%
Denmark	97	33.6%	7848	0.8%	Maryland	386	54.3%
Hungary	52	23.8%	8639	0.9%	Delaware	344	64.2%
Norway	43	57.9%	7470	0.7%	USAc	304	53.6%
Australia	4	29.3%	7436	0.7%	Mississippi	219	50.7%
Singapore	4	11.1%	2745	0.3%	Georgia	178	51.1%
Hong Kong	0.5	0.0%	9737	1.0%	Washington	143	61.1%
					California	97	42.1%
					Kentucky	88	56.1%
					Texas	54	45.7%
					Tennessee	52	35.4%
					Arkansas	39	42.0%

(continued)

Table 1.1 (continued)

Nation	COVID-19 death rate per million population, May 27 2020	Deaths in nursing homes as a % of total COVID-related deaths, May 22 2020	Long term residential care beds per million persons	Long term residential care beds as a % of total population	US State	COVID-19 death rate per million population, May 27 2020	Deaths in nursing homes as a % of total COVID-related deaths, May 12 2020
					Oregon	35	59.3%

Source: The Foundation for Research on Equal Opportunity (FREEOP), Reported Deaths from COVID-19 in Long Term Care Facilities, Deaths reported by May 22, 2020; UK deaths in nursing homes: Jeremy Hunt, Chair of the British Parliament's Health and Social Care Committee (HSCC); OECD Stat, Long-Term Care Resources and Utilisation, Beds in residential long-term care facilities, 2016 (Germany, 2017; Denmark, 2011); Singapore Ministry of Health, Resources & Statistics, Beds In Inpatient Facilities and Places In Non-Residential Long-Term Care Facilities; Ernest Chui, Long-Term Care Policy in Hong Kong: Challenges and Future Directions, Home Health Care Services Quarterly, 30(3):119–32, July 2011

[a]Estimated by Jeremy Hunt, Chair of the British Parliament's Health and Social Care Committee. Booth, R. "MP's hear why Hong Kong had no Covid-19 care home deaths", The Guardian, May 20, 2020
[b]Stockholm region
[c]Excludes New York State as the state classified many nursing home deaths as hospital deaths

died after being infected with the virus would have died in 2020 in any event.[7] Such deaths should not show-up in statistical reporting as excess deaths—that is as deaths over and above the expected national median for a given week. So it is statistically possible to filter such persons out of the picture of mortality by looking at excess deaths that occurred above the weekly national norm. In March, April and May 2020, many countries confronting COVID-19 did not register significant or even any increases in excess deaths—i.e. deaths above the norm. Yet other countries did (Table 1.2). This is puzzling. Why did some COVID-affected countries experience much higher than normal mortality rates while others did not?

As Table 1.3 indicates, COVID-19 was associated with a wide span of rates of fatality between countries. As we will see later on, the same thing applied between regions in the United States and Canada. This suggests that, in addition to the biochemical characteristics and behaviour of the virus, there are social reasons or social contexts that explain—or partly explain—the significant variations in the number of fatalities per capita between nations and regions. Lower and higher national and regional rates of death reflect a range of R_E and infection fatality rates. The variation of fatalities per capita between and within nations is striking.

In the case of COVID-19, a vaccine in 2020 was unlikely to happen. This did not mean that it would not or could not happen. Just that the probability of it happening was low. Vaccines are slow to develop and test—twelve to eighteen months from March 2020 was the most common optimistic timeline given for a COVID-19 vaccine. It was also widely observed that a vaccine might never eventuate, or it might be many years away, or it might only protect some people. For all its resources, pharmaceutical science has not had much success over decades in creating antiviral vaccines. It took 47 years to develop a vaccine for polio, 46 years for measles, 35 years for yellow fever, 22 years for the Hepatovirus A, and 17 years for the Hepatitis B virus. One in ninety antiviral vaccine projects fail. In April 2020 there were eighty COVID-19 vaccine projects under way around the world (Swan 2020, April 13). By May that number had risen to 100. With that degree of investment of resources and time, it was plausible to think that a vaccine would be produced. Yet that was not guaranteed—due to the very high failure rate of such projects. Hope is not a scientific methodology.

In any event vaccines do not always provide comprehensive immunity. The efficacy of seasonal flu vaccines varies from year to year. The elderly—the principal COVID risk group—often respond less well to vaccines. If not

Table 1.2 European mortality, excess deaths, z-scores, March–April 2020

Week	Dates	England	Wales	Scotland	France	Germany[a]	Belgium	Spain	Norway	Sweden	Italy	Switzerland
Week 11	March 9–15	NE	NE	NE	NE	NE	NE	LE	NE	NE	ME	NE
Week 12	March 16–22	ME	NE	NE	ME	NE	ME	VH	NE	NE	VH	ME
Week 13	March 23–March 29	EH	ME	ME	VH	NE	EH	EH	NE	ME	EH	ME
Week 14	March 30–April 5	EH	VH	VH	EH	NE	EH	EH	NE	VH	EH	VH
Week 15	April 6–April 12	EH	EH	EH	EH	NE	EH	EH	NE	VH	EH	HE
Week 16	April 13–April 20	EH	ME	VH	LE	NE	ME	ME	NE	LE	ME	ME
Week 17	April 21–April 28	EH	VH	VH	LE	NE	VH	ME	NE	HE	ME	LE
Week 18	April 29–May 5	EH	NE	HE	NE	NE	ME	NE	NE	ME	NE	NE

Week	Dates	Denmark	Austria	Hungary	Greece	Portugal	Netherlands	Ireland	N Ireland	Finland	Estonia
Week 11	March 9–15	NE	NE	NE	NE	NE	LE	NE	NE	NE	NE
Week 12	March 16–22	NE	LE	NE	NE	LE	ME	NE	NE	NE	NE
Week 13	March 23–March 29	NE	NE	NE	NE	LE	EH	NE	NE	NE	NE
Week 14	March 30–April 5	NE	LE	NE	NE	ME	EH	NE	ME	NE	NE
Week 15	April 6–April 12	LE	NE	NE	NE	ME	EH	NE	ME	NE	NE
Week 16	April 13–April 20	NE	NE	NE	NE	LE	HE	NE	NE	NE	NE
Week 17	April 21–April 28	NE	NE	NE	NE	LE	VH	NE	ME	NE	NE
Week 18	April 29–May 5	NE	NE	NE	NE	NE	NE	NE	NE	NE	NE

Z-scores: NE = no excess less than 2; LE = low excess 2–4; ME = moderate excess 4–7; HE = high excess 7–10; VH = very high excess 10–15; EH = extremely high >15

Source: Euro Mono, Mortality Monitoring in Europe, Map of z-scores by country

Note: A z-score indicates how far from a mean a data point is

[a] Berlin and Hesse only

Table 1.3 COVID-19, selected countries, deaths per million population and contextual factors, May 27, 2020

Country	First confirmed case 2020	Days from first confirmed case to day of peak daily deaths	Total Covid-19 deaths	Population	COVID-19-related deaths per million pop	Median age of the population	Total annual deaths, latest available[a]	Annual deaths per million pop
Spain	February 1	66	27,117	46,754,778	580	42.7	422,568	9038
United Kingdom	January 31	69	37,048	67,886,011	546	40.5	602,781	8879
Italy	January 31	57	32,955	60,461,826	545	45.5	646,048	10,685
France	January 24	64	28,530	65,273,511	437	41.4	544,618	8344
Sweden	January 31	82	4125	10,099,265	408	41.2	91,071	9018
Netherlands	February 27	41	5856	17,134,872	342	42.6	148,997	8696
United States	January 24	58	100,572	331,002,651	304	38.1	2,712,630	8195
Switzerland	February 25	40	1915	8,654,622	221	42.4	67,606	7812
Canada	January 25	98	6639	37,742,154	176	42.4	252,338	6686
Germany	January 27	73	8498	83,783,942	101	47.1	925,200	11,043
Denmark	February 27	38	563	5,792,202	97	42.2	52,224	9016
Hungary	March 4	46	459	9,660,351	52	42.3	127,053	13,152
Norway	February 27	54	235	5,421,241	43	39.2	40,686	7505
Japan	January 16	86	846	126,476,461	6.7	47.3	1,290,444	10,203
South Korea	January 20	65	269	51,269,185	5.2	41.8	275,895	5381
Australia	January 25	73	103	25,499,884	4.0	38.7	159,052	6237
Singapore	January 23	[b]	23	5,850,342	3.9	34.6	18,640	3186
China	November 17, 2019	[c]	4634	1,439,323,776	3.2	37.4	9,980,000	6934
Hong Kong	January 23	[b]	4	7,496,981	0.5	43.5	46,757	6237

(*continued*)

Table 1.3 (continued)

Country	First confirmed case 2020	Days from first confirmed case to day of peak daily deaths	Total Covid-19 deaths	Population	COVID-19-related deaths per million pop	Median age of the population	Total annual deaths, latest available[a]	Annual deaths per million pop
Taiwan	January 21	[b]	7	23,816,775	0.3	40.7	172,418	7239

Data sources: Worldometer Coronavirus countries data https://www.worldometers.info/; Worldometer Countries in the world by population (2020) based on United Nations 2019 Population Division estimates; Median age by country, CIA World Factbook 2018; World Health Organization Morality Database; Worldlife expectancy, Influenza and pneumonia death rate per 100,000, based on World Health Organization Age-adjusted death rate estimates, 2017; China National Bureau of Statistics 2019; Taiwan Ministry of Health and Welfare, 2016; Worldometer, Coronavirus, Daily deaths by nation; UK NHS COVID-19 daily deaths summary May 3 2020

[a]Latest available figures from World Health Organization Mortality Database
[b]Too few deaths to identify a peak
[c]Change in data collection recording makes identification of peak uncertain

a vaccine then what? One option in lieu of a vaccine is community immunity ("herd immunity")—when enough healthy members of the population are exposed to the virus without getting seriously ill or dying or even knowing they have been exposed. Susceptibility to a virus varies. It may be conditioned by an adaptive immunity built up in a population through exposure to an earlier comparable virus. The alternatives to herd immunity included social distancing, that is, creating sufficient physical distance between people (limiting close contact), and fine-tuning environmental (including sanitation and ventilation) conditions to reduce the communicability of the disease. A further option was all of the above combined. In a combined scenario, those at low risk (the young) carry the burden of herd immunity while those at high risk, the elderly, are physically distanced.[8]

Human populations naturally wish to acquire immunity—however it is obtained—for a very simple reason. A small percentage of persons who fall sick from exposure to a viral pathogen will fall seriously or critically ill from the virus and some will die from it. As in the case of COVID-19 a critical illness can mean not only death but long-term damage to the body.[9] Like other viral pathogens, COVID-19 has an infection fatality rate (IFR). This is the percentage of those who get infected who die. In the case of COVID-19, like the R_0 and R_E, it is better to think of the IFR of the virus not as a single number but rather as a range of numbers. The pattern of deaths per capita that occurred during the months of January through May 2020 indicated that COVID-19 was associated with a considerable range of different infection fatality rates in different countries, regions and cities. In short, a single IFR for COVID-19 did not apply uniformly across the world. Heterogeneity rather than homogeneity characterised the impact of the virus.

Anthony Fauci, the director of the US National Institute of Allergy and Infectious Diseases, in an editorial for *The New England Journal of Medicine* published online on February 28, 2020, said that, among diagnosed cases, ultimately the consequences of COVID-19 will be "more akin to those of a severe seasonal influenza (which has a case fatality rate of approximately 0.1%) or a pandemic influenza (similar to those in 1957 and 1968) rather than a disease similar to SARS or MERS, which have had case fatality rates of 9 to 10% and 36%, respectively" (Fauci et al. 2020, February 26). Thirteen days later on March 11, giving evidence before the US Congress' House Committee on Oversight and Government Reform, Fauci estimated that the mortality rate of the virus was at around 1% "which means it is ten times more lethal than the seasonal flu" (Facher 2020, March 11).

The American Centers for Disease Control (CDC) similarly see-sawed. In March the CDC estimated an infection fatality rate (IFR) of 0.8% of all persons infected, not just diagnosed cases. In late May in a revised estimate it calculated a case fatality rate (CFR) of 0.4% together with a rate of asymptotic infections of 35%. An infection fatality rate of 0.25% can be inferred from those figures. The infection fatality rate for the seasonal flu in 2018–2019 in the United States was just under 0.1% (based on an estimated 34,000 related deaths among 35 million flu cases during that year).[10]

Estimates in early April of the virus' IFR ranged from 0.01% to 0.36% including random-sample research conducted in Germany and Iceland (Table 1.4). As of May 20 2020 34 serological studies of the virus had been undertaken.[11] The median average IFR across these studies was 0.37%. The infection fatality rate calculated on the basis of different individual studies ranged from 1.15% (Milan) to 0% (San Migue, Colorado). John Ioannidis reviewed 12 of those studies (excluding those with a low sample size and other prohibitive design features). Of that cohort of 12, the inferred infection fatality rates ranged from 0.03% to 0.50% and the corrected values ranged from 0.02% to 0.40%.[12] Seven of the 12 inferred IFRs were in the range 0.07% to 0.20% (the corrected IFRs were in the range of 0.06% to 0.16%) which, Ioannidis observed, were similar to the IFR values of a seasonal influenza. Three of the values were modestly higher; one value was lower than this range. It should also be noted that serological tests identify anti-bodies produced by B cell and mucosal immune reactions. However seronegative persons (those who test negative for anti-bodies) may test positive for T cells. One study of May 2020 Swedish blood donors reported that almost twice the number of the donors had generated memory T cell responses compared to antibodies (Sekine et al. 2020).

In one important respect, virus behaviour is predictable. As William Farr discovered in the nineteenth century, viral infections expand and decline at a bell-curve shaped rate.[13] Slowly at first, followed by a quick-paced rise upwards, then a cap, then a quick-paced decline and finally (slowly again) a taper until the virus fades out.[14] The curve upwards and downwards can be relatively steep or comparatively gentle. Nations or regions that are successful (for whatever reason) in moderating the bell curve reduce the R_E number (the number of persons an infected person will infect in practice) as well as the fatality rate among infected people. Given the history of viruses there is no guarantee that the bell curve pattern of infection will not recur in the form of a series of bell curves or "waves" of infection, though this does not always occur.

Table 1.4 COVID-19 infection fatality rates (IFR) and projected resulting deaths among infected national populations

Country	Population, 2019	60% of population infected ['herd immunity' threshold]	*If: the IFR assumption*					
			Baseline: University of Bonn 17 April estimated IFR for Gangelt Germany	Baseline: P. Simon April 10 estimated IFR for Iceland	Baseline: Oxford Centre for Evidence Based Medicine April 9 estimated IFR range for Iceland		Total annual deaths, 2015	Deaths, coronary heart disease, 2017
			COVID-19 infection fatality rate 0.36%	COVID-19 infection fatality rate 0.04%	COVID-19 infection fatality rate 0.19%	COVID-19 infection fatality rate 0.01%		
			Then: projected deaths per nation					
Australia	25,203,000	15,121,800	54,438	6049	28,731	1512	159,052	23,153
United Kingdom	65,650,000	39,390,000	141,804	15,756	74,841	3939	602,781	75,426
United States	328,200,000	196,920,000	708,912	78,768	374,148	19,692	2,712,630	479,223
Sweden	10,230,000	6,138,000	22,097	2455	11,662	614	91,071	17,223
Italy	60,360,000	36,216,000	130,378	14,486	68,810	3622	646,048	108,924

Sources: WHO Mortality Database; WorldLifeExpectancy data based on WHO age-adjusted death rate estimates, 2017; Hendrik Streeck, Covid-19 case cluster study, Heinsberg district Germany, University of Bonn; Estimating COVID-19 Infection Fatality Rates (IFR) 9 April 2020, Centre for Evidence-Based Medicine, Global Covid-19 Case Fatality Rates, 21st April 2020; Gudbjartsson, D.F. et al., Spread of SARS CoV-2 in the Icelandic Population, New England Journal of Medicine, April 16, 2020; Simon, P., Robust Estimation of Infection Fatality Rates during the Early Phase of a Pandemic, medRxiv preprint, April 10 2020

(*continued*)

Table 1.4 (continued)

Note: The infection fatality rate of seasonal flu strains is around 0.1% https://www.cdc.gov/flu/about/burden/index.html; the Gangelt study was a random sample of 1000 residents; as of March 29 deCode Genetics in Iceland had tested 5571 Icelanders on a quasi-random basis. The Gudbjartsson et al. Icelandic study included a targeted testing population [9199 persons with symptoms or who had travelled to high-risk countries or who had been in contact with infected persons; testing by the National University Iceland Hospital; 2.9% of Iceland's population], 10,979 persons who were issued with an open invitation to test, and a random sampling of 2283 persons [3.7% of Iceland's population; testing carried out by deCode Genetics]. As of April 4 2020, 0.8% in the open-invitation group and 0.6% in the random population group tested positive for the virus. Of the targeted population of high-risk individuals, 13.3% tested positive for the virus. The Oxford Centre for Evidence-Based Medicine estimated from this data an IFR for Iceland in the range of 0.01–0.19%. P. Simon estimated from the epidemiological data an IFR of 0.040% compared to his mathematically-derived estimate of 0.05–0.13% with a median estimate of 0.10%

What explains the variation in the R_E number and the infection fatality rate within and between nations and regions? What explains the large range in the incidence of deaths per capita between (say) Italy and Taiwan (Table 1.3)? Why does one society have over five hundred deaths per million population while another society has a handful of deaths per million population? During the COVID-19 episode explanations multiplied. They included climate (temperature), ICUs (intensive care units) per capita, the percentage of persons in single households, the percentage of persons in multi-generational households, air quality by country, the death rate per capita from influenza and pneumonia, the national median age, and the rate of smoking per country.[15] The explanations went like this: COVID-19 survives a shorter period of time in sunlight;[16] single persons are more socially isolated; youthful populations are less at risk; multi-generational families are more likely to transmit the virus from the young to the most-at-risk elderly populations. In addition, because COVID-19 attacks the respiratory system, there are several respiratory-related possible causes: air pollution and smoking. The incidence of influenza is a proxy for the state of the respiratory health of a susceptible population. As is evident from Table 1.5, 1.6 and 1.7, there is no correlation between COVID-19 deaths per capita and these factors except intergenerational contact.[17]

1.3 INTERPERSONAL DISTANCE

A lot of explanations for the variable impact of COVID-19 ignored the most elementary fact about the virus. It is passed on by close contact between persons. The virus is transmitted via droplets or aerosol particles. A droplet or particle containing the virus passes from one person to another person (or persons) who are in close physical contact with the first person.[18] The second person draws it in through the mouth, nose or eyes. As we'll see in a moment, close contact—the proximity of one person to another—is not only a physical or bio-medical phenomenon. It is also a social one.

In late March 2020 researchers from Bonn University undertook a preliminary virological study of Gangelt in Germany, a town hit hard by COVID-19 (Streeck et al. 2020, April 9).[19] They could find no evidence of the transmission of the virus in supermarkets, restaurants or hairdressing salons. Rather, they concluded, major outbreaks of the virus were the result of close-packed get-togethers that took place over extended periods of time.[20] Outbreaks stemmed from tightly-packed events such as after-ski parties with people pressed together in close quarters for a sustained

Table 1.5 COVID-19 conjectured contextual factors: which, if any, factors correlate with country deaths per million?

Country	COVID-19-related deaths per million pop, May 27 2020	ICUs per 100,000 population[a]	Average annual temperature degrees C	Population per square km of largest city	CV tests per million performed by March 13-20	% of single person households[b]	% of 'other' [not couple, single parent or single person] households[b]	Inter-generational close contact, care for parents during the last 12 months, percent per country	Air quality by largest city, unless noted, Air Quality Index, 0 = best quality	Influenza and pneumonia death rate per million 2017	International visitors [business, tourism, personal] to number one destination city, millions 2016	Median age of the population	Rate of smoking per population
Spain	580	8.2–9.7	13.3	5200	642	23.19	10.62	10%	24	102	8.2	42.7	20%
United Kingdom	546	3.5–7.4	8.45	5100	952	30.58	10.12	10%	29	230	19.88	40.5	19%
Italy	545		13.45	2950	3422	31.08	8.61	4%	132[d]	82	7.65	45.5	24%
France	437		10.7	3550	563	33.79	4.81	4%	41	141	8	41.4	28%
Sweden	408		2.1	2700	1416	36.22	5.02	6%		156	2.08	41.2	21%
Netherlands	342		9.25	4908	350	36.38	1.71		27	146	8	42.6	25%
United States	304	20–31.7	8.55	2050	314	26.74	15.29		4	149	12.75	38.1	17%
Switzerland	221		5.5	4700	462	36.98	3.04	5%	55[e]	102	2.24	42.2	23%
Canada	176	13.5	-5.35	2650	3000	27.58	6.09		33	93	4.52	42.4	15%
Germany	101		8.5	3750	1993	37.27	5.52	6%	30	109	4.94	47.1	30%
Denmark	97	6.7–8.9	7.5	1850	1852	37.48	6.16	4%		171	1.63	42.2	17%
Hungary	52		9.75	2550	311	32.08	8.88		78	61	3.36	42.3	28%
Norway	43		1.5	3300	8067	39.58	4.68		8	196		39.2	22%
Japan	6.7	7.9	11.15	4750	276	34.45	16.16		33	345	11.7	47.3	22%
South Korea	5		11.5	16,700	6176	23.90	14.50		122	198	10.2	41.8	27%
Australia	4.0	8.0–8.9	21.65	2100	4456	23.90	8.70		13	97	3.7	38.7	15%
Singapore	3.9		26.45	8350	6495				53	701	12.11	34.6	17%
China	3.2	2.8–4.6	6.95	11,500					128[f]	147	6.12	37.4	25%
Hong Kong	0.5		22.6	6659	703						8.37	43.5	
Taiwan	0.3		22	15,200	898				62		7.35	40.7	

Sources: Meghan Prin and Hannah Wunsch, International comparisons of intensive care: informing outcomes and improving standards, Current opinion in critical care. 2012 Dec; 18(6): 700–706, Table 1; CityMayors Statistics, The largest cities in the world by land area, population and density; World Population Review; Ourworldindata, coronavirus-testing-source-data, country statistics and sources; Financial Times, How Singapore waged war on coronavirus, March 22, 2020; OECD Family Database, SF1.1: Family size and household composition, Table SF1.1.A. Types of household, 2011, Distribution (%) of households by household type; Martina Brandt, Klaus Haberkern and Marc Szydlik, Intergenerational Help and Care in Europe, European Sociological Review, 25:5, 2009, 585–601, Fig. 2 Care for parents during the last 12 months [data from The Survey of Health, Ageing and Retirement (SHARE), 11 European countries surveyed]; IQAir, Air quality and pollution city ranking, April 2020; worldlifeexpectancy.com, cause-of-death, influenza-pneumonia by-country based on World Health Organization data, 2017; Mastercard Global Destinations Cities Index, 2016; World Population Review, Countries, Smoking Rates by Country 2020

Note: The correlation coefficients of explanatory variables to the outcome variable of COVID deaths per capita: temperature [weak 0.25], urban density [weak 0.37], tests performed [moderate 0.47], solo households [weak 0.12], other households [weak 0.29], air quality [weak 0.1], flu deaths per capita [weak 0.30], international visitors [weak 0.24], median age [weak 0.17] and smoking rate [weak 0.007]; inter-generational contact [moderate 0.62]

[a]ICUs are defined by countries in many different ways. These estimates, from Prin and Wunsch (2012), accordingly involve different definitions of ICU beds

[b]OECD-32 average: 30.56% for single person households; 9.81% for 'other' households

[c]These are the number of formally registered flu and pneumonia-related deaths; estimated annual deaths associated with flu and pneumonia but not formally certified as such are substantially higher in number

[d]Milan

[e]Bern

[f]Wuhan

Table 1.6 Air pollution by major COVID-19 affected cities, 2016

City	PM2.5^a Annual mean, ug/m^3, 2016
Wuhan	57
Daegu, S Korea	42
Madrid	10
New York	7
Detroit	8
Denver	8
Milan	27
London	12
New Orleans	8

Top-50 world's most polluted cities, 2019 average PM2.5

Number one most polluted: Ghaziabad, India, 110.2 PM2.5

Number fifty most polluted: Bhiwani, India 61.6 PM2.5

Sources: WHO air quality database, 2016 data unless otherwise stated; World most polluted cities 2019 (PM2.5), IQAir. New Orleans air pollution data 2014

^{a}Atmospheric particulate matter (PM) that have a diameter of less than 2.5 micro-metres

Table 1.7 Air passengers by major COVID-19 affected cities, 2018

City	Airline passengers, 2018	City population, 2019	Annual passengers per city resident
COVID-19 Hotspot cities			
Daegu, S Korea	2,530,000	2,460,000	1.0
Madrid	57,891,340	5,567,000	10.4
New York	141,964,323	19,354,922	7.3
Detroit	35,236,676	3,522,206	10.0
Denver	64,494,613	2,787,266	23.1
Milan	24,600,000	2,945,000	8.4
London	177,276,807	8,567,000	20.7
New Orleans	13,100,000	1,029,123	12.7
Comparator cities			
Sydney	44,400,000	4,630,000	9.6
Singapore	65,628,000	5,183,700	12.7
Hong Kong	74,517,402	7,206,000	10.3
Los Angeles	109,825,171	12,815,475	8.6
Stockholm	26,800,000	1,264,000	21.2

Sources: Airports Council International, World Airport Traffic Report, 2018; Simple Maps, World Cities Database, 2019. Supplementary air traffic data: Daegu 2016, New Orleans 2018, Sydney 2018, Detroit 2018, Milan 2018, Stockholm 2018

period of time. Football crowds and carnival celebrants were also directly connected to outbreaks.[21] Whether the relevant transmissions occurred outdoors or in related celebrations in bars or in packed transport going home—crowded enclosed spaces—was not established.[22] Chinese research (below) though suggested that transmission occured mostly in enclosed spaces. The Bonn researchers could detect the virus when they swabbed tactile surfaces such as remote controls, washbasins, mobile phones, toilets and door handles. However they only detected RNA, the ribonucleic acid (genetic information) of "dead" viruses. As the lead virologist observed in reported remarks: a door handle could only be infectious if someone has actually coughed in their hand and then reached for it. "After that, you have to reach for the door handle yourself and touch your face" (Anon 2020, April 2).

In China, researchers studying the transmission of the virus also raised doubts that supermarkets, restaurants and hairdressers were significant locations of transmission (Qian et al. 2020, April 7). The Chinese researchers looked at outbreaks involving three or more secondary cases in 320 municipalities in China. The study excluded Hubei province where the virus pandemic began as well as Beijing, Shanghai, and Guangzhou. From a total of 7324 cases and 318 clusters tabulated for the study, the researchers found that 254 (79.9%) of the outbreak clusters occurred in a home (one in a villa; all others in apartments), 108 (34.0%) occurred in a transport location, 14 (4.4%) at a restaurant or other food venue, 7 (2.2%) at an entertainment venue, 7 (2.2%) at a shopping location (shopping mall and supermarket), and 26 (8.1%) at a miscellaneous location (e.g., hospital, hotel room, unspecified community venue, power plant). All of the cluster outbreaks identified from municipal data occurred in indoor (enclosed space) locations.

The research drew on municipal data from January 4 to February 11 2020. Wuhan, the centre of China's mass outbreak, was locked down on January 23. Chinese New Year 2020 ran from Saturday January 25 to February 8 so the data was necessarily skewed against workplace locations for virus transmission and skewed in favour of family travel for Chinese New Year. After the January 23 shutdown of Wuhan, Chinese across the country began voluntarily staying home. Nonetheless it is notable that, at a busy shopping, eating-out and public entertainment time of year, virus transmission mostly occurred between family members, relatives, and socially-connected individuals and *not* between socially-unconnected individuals (strangers). Among the 318 cluster outbreaks, 129 (40%) involved only family members, 133 (41.8%) involved family relatives, and 29 (9%) involved socially-connected individuals. In contrast only 24 (7.5%) involved socially un-connected individuals (strangers).

One of the earliest studies of transmission outside of China, an American study (from March 6, 2020) monitored 445 persons who had come into contact with 10 US cases of confirmed travel-related COVID. Four percent of the 445 were household members. The rest were community contacts with more than 10 minutes of physical contact within a proximity of 6 feet as well as community contacts in health care settings and health care workers. Of all of these, two only—both of them household members— tested positive to COVID (Burke et al. 2020, March 6). Subsequently a review was conducted of the (then) first known person in Illinois in the US to be infected with COVID—a woman in her sixties who had travelled from China in January. This March 13 study monitored 347 contacts of hers and her husband who also became infected. Of those contacts, none contracted the virus except her husband. The conclusion of the study was that "person-to-person transmission of SARS-CoV-2 occurred between two people with prolonged, unprotected exposure while Patient 1 was symptomatic" (Ghinai et al. 2020, March 13, p. 1137).

A study of close contacts in Ningbo city in China, published on March 26 2020 reported that of 2147 close contacts tracked and investigated, 6.1% were infected by contact (Chen et al. 2020, March 4). Of that number, 22.31% were friends, 18.01% were family members and 4.73% were relatives. Close contacts of medical staff were not infected. Living with an infected person (13.26%), taking the same transportation together (11.91%), and dining together (7.18%) were high risk factors for infection. 1.94% were cross-infections in hospitals. From January 14 to February 12 2020, the Shenzhen Center for Disease Control and Prevention identified 391 COVID cases and 1286 close contacts (Bi et al. 2020, April 27). The observed reproduction number (R) was 0·4. The cases were older than the general population (mean age 45 years). Household contacts and those travelling with a case were at higher risk of infection than other close contacts. 77 (91%) of the 84 infected contacts were associated with household contact (Bi et al. 2020, April 27, Table 3). The household secondary attack rate was 11·2%, that is, fewer than one in six contacts.[23]

A study was undertaken between January 15 and March 18 in Taiwan of 100 cases and their 2761 close contacts (Cheng et al. 2020, May 1). 5.5% of the contacts were household contacts, 2.8% were non-household family contacts, and 25.3% were health care contacts. 23 secondary cases were found. 6.6% of household contacts contracted the disease along with 6.5% of non-household family, 0.85% of healthcare workers and 0.054% of others. Secondary infection was higher among persons aged 40 to 59 years (1.25%) and those aged 60 years and older (0.9%) than the 20–39 (0.68%) or 0–19 (0.35%) age groups (Cheng et al. 2020, May 1, Table 2).

A Guangzhou China study of contact tracing looked at 212 primary cases involving 137 secondary or tertiary cases and 1938 uninfected close contacts. Comparing household and non-household contacts, the overall non-primary attack rates—that is, the percentages of at-risk populations during a specified time interval—were 12.6% and 3.06% respectively. Households were much more conducive to transmission. So much so that the Guangzhou study surmised that "within-household transmission might have contributed substantially to the continued rise in cases in China even after the introduction of nationally enforced restrictions on human movement. Home isolation/quarantine of people with an exposure history or mild symptoms is frequently recommended as a disease control measure in countries with COVID-19 outbreaks, but such restrictions likely have limited or no effect on family transmission" (Jing et al. 2020, April 15). A March 30 2020 study, this one an analysis of literature published between December 2019 and March 2020, looked at 31 household transmission clusters from China, Singapore, South Korea, Japan, and Iran. It concluded that of these clusters only 9.7% (3/31) had a child source. The view of the study was that "while SARS-CoV-2 can cause mild disease in children, the data... suggests that children have not played a substantive role in the intra-household transmission of SARS-CoV-2" (Zhu et al. 2020, March 30).

What these figures underlined is the degree to which COVID-19 is a disease of social proximity or close contact. Families (adult members) and homes (including nursing homes and families travelling together) figure prominently in the transmission of the virus because they are relationships and locations of close contact. The crowding of persons in enclosed social spaces has a similar effect. Early large outbreaks of the virus were associated with close contact in crowded charismatic church assemblies and cruise ships.[24]

What if the pattern that applied at a micro-social level also applied at the macro-social level? The virus transmits—or doesn't transmit—subject to how intensely physically-close individuals touch each other, breath-on each other or in some way communicate microscopic sprays to each other. How does this operate on a large social scale—at the level of nations or regions? Is relative physical distance something that not only occurs between dyads and triads and small groups of human beings in close or crowded contact but also is manifest on a large social scale involving millions of people?

The anthropologist Edward T. Hall introduced the idea of proxemics to the social sciences in the 1960s (Hall 1966). Proxemics—and related to it haptics (touch)—is the study of personal space. This is the space that persons normally allow for in their interactions with others—families, friends, acquaintances and strangers. What this research over the years has shown is that personal space varies by nation and region—considerably. A number of serious studies have measured habitual physical distance between nationalities and between denizens of regions within nations. The discipline of inter-cultural business communication studies has also produced a large literature based on accumulated observation and reporting of national personal spatial habits—a subject of some importance when Americans and Japanese or Swedes and Italians do business together.

Table 1.8 compares death rates per capita connected to COVID-19 with national interpersonal spatial habits. Interpersonal distances vary between nations. This is true of interactions with strangers, acquaintances and families. Table 1.9 illustrates the difference between France and Germany. Those relative distances mirror the rates of COVID-related deaths per capita to a significant degree as does the propensity of national subjects to touch each other, as do meeting-and-greeting conventions— notably so when the causal effects of all of these traits combine (Table 1.8). The kiss-on-the-cheek versus the handshake versus the bow-nod greeting all imply relative degrees of social distance that mirror the relative spread and impact of COVID-19 between nations.

What applies on a national level is replicated, in a fractal manner, on a regional level, as Tables 1.10 and 1.11 illustrate.[25] A high-contact culture is a culture in which habitual everyday physical interactions between people are close by comparison to low-contact cultures where physical distance is, as a matter of habit, greater. The degree of distancing is culturally-specific, the product of the long history of cultural ancestry. The habit of distancing is formed early in childhood. Three cases are examined in detail here: the United States, Canada and Italy. French and Italian cultural ancestry is used as a proxy for high-contact culture in North America. In the case of the United States, the incidence by region of the "un-inhibited" personality type is also used as a proxy for close-contact. In the case of Italy (Table 1.11), the proxy for a high-contact culture is a

Table 1.8 Preferred interpersonal social distancing and COVID-19, selected countries

Countries	COVID-19 deaths per million pop, May 27 2020	Social Distance (Stranger) cm	Personal Distance (Acquaintance) cm	Intimate Distance (Close Person) cm	Average distance cm	Average distance in arm-length	Intimate distance in arm-length	Mean number of body parts touched in public personal interaction	Conventional greeting: cheek kissing (CK), hand shaking (HS), bowing/nodding (BN)	Social Distance (Stranger), seated, mean head-to-head proximity cm	Social Distance (Stranger), mean torso-to-torso proximity in busy public spaces cm
Spain	580	91	74	57	74	1.61	1.24		CK		
United Kingdom	546	98	82	56	79	1.71	1.22	5.67	HS	45	39
English											27
Scottish											26
Irish											
Italy	545	95	68	45	69	1.51	0.98		CK		36
France	437							4.75	CK	60	36
Netherlands	342								CK	66	35
United States	304	95	68	50	71	1.54	1.09	6.72	HS		
Switzerland	221	110	93	73	92	2.00	1.59	4	CK		
Canada	176	100	88	73	87	1.89	1.59		HS		
Germany	101	95	64	42	67	1.46	0.91	6	HS		
Denmark	97							8	HS		
Hungary	52	130	108	95	111	2.41	2.07	6	CK		
Norway	43	102	72	37	70	1.53	0.80		HS		
Japan	7							2	BN		
South Korea	5	108	84	65	86	1.86	1.41	0.91	BN		
Australia	4				83[a]	1.80			HS		
China	3.2	115	83	58	85	1.86	1.26	1.33[b]	BN/HS		
Hong Kong	0.5	112	87	69	89	1.94	1.50	1.33[b]	HS		
Taiwan	0.3							1.33[b]	BN		

Sources: Sorokowska, A., et al. (2017) Preferred interpersonal distances: a global comparison. Journal of Cross-Cultural Psychology, 48 (4). pp. 577–592; McDaniel E. & Andersen, P.A. International Patterns of Interpersonal Tactile Communication: A Field Study, Journal of Nonverbal Behavior 22(1), Spring 1998; Moss, T. A Guide to Kissing Etiquette Around the World, Conde Nast Traveller, October 18, 2017; eDiplomat, Cultural Etiquette, Meeting and Greeting; Remland, M.S., et al. (1991) Proxemic and Haptic Behavior in Three European Countries, Journal of Nonverbal Behavior 15(4), Table 1; Remland, M.S., et al. (1995) Interpersonal Distance, Body Orientation, and Touch: Effects of Culture, Gender, and Age, The Journal of Social Psychology, 135(3), 281–297

(continued)

Table 1.8 (continued)

Note: Coefficient correlates of the explanatory proxemic and haptic variables with the outcome variable (COVID mortality per capita): stranger, personal and intimate distances combined [strong 0.79], body touching [moderate 0.61], greeting styles [moderate 0.64]; when all the explanatory variables are analysed together, the relationship is a very strong one [0.96].

Note: Average distance of arm from shoulder to finger-tip: 46 cm

[a] Median distance estimated based on Noesjirwan, J., Contrasting Cultural Patterns of Interpersonal Closeness in Doctors' Waiting Rooms in Sydney and Jakarta, Journal of Cross-Cultural Psychology, September 1977, Vol.8(3), 357–368

[b] Combines China, Hong Kong and Taiwan

Table 1.9 Europe, comparative locations, preferred interpersonal social distancing, 2014, centimetres

	Leipzig, Germany					Lyon, France				
Relationship	Formal Public	Casual Public	Party	Formal Private	Formal Casual	Formal Public	Casual Public	Party	Formal Private	Formal Casual
Spouse/Significant Other	40–60	20–60	40–60	40–60	0–40	20–30	0–20	0–25	25–30	0–20
Family Member	20–60	20–60	20–60	20–60	20–60	20–30	0–20	0–25	25–35	0–25
Very Close Friend	40–60	20–60	20–60	40–60	20–60	0–15	0–10	0–10	0–15	0–10
Friend	~60	~50	~50	~60	~50	15–30	10–20	10–20	20–40	10–20
Group of Friends	~50	~50	~50	~50	~50	5–10	5–10	5–10	5–10	5–10
Acquaintance	60–90	60–90	60–90	60–90	60–90	20–40	10–20	10–20	20–40	10–20
Stranger	60–90	60–90	60–90	60–90	60–90	100+	100+	100+	100+	100+
Facility Staff	60–90	60–90	60–90	60–90	60–90	SH	SH	SH	SH	SH

SH = depends on status hierarchy

Source: Joel Vervoort, Paige Arding, Mark Lasia, Chukwunonso Bernard-Oti; Proxemics Across Europe, 2014, https://prezi.com/ulqcwyickq5n/proxemics-across-europe/ Data based on interviews with subjects, with a bias toward younger adult subjects. The study was undertaken, as many proxemic studies are, by marketing and business communication professionals

Table 1.10 High-contact culture: US and Canada

State	COVID-19 death rate per million population, May 27 2020	% of population with Italian cultural ancestry [highest: 6% and over][a,b]	% of population who report Italian cultural ancestry first or second in the American Community Survey [highest states: 16–19%, lowest states: 0–4%][a]	% of population who report French cultural ancestry first or second in the American Community Survey [highest states: 8–16%; lowest states: 0–2%][a]	Uninhibited personality type by state [high incidence: 5 low incidence: -5][a]	Urban population, % of total population, 2010
New York	1514	6% and over	12–16%	2–4%	5	87.9%
New Jersey	1261	6% and over	16–19%	0–2%	3	94.7%
Connecticut	1057	6% and over	16–19%	4–6%	3	88.0%
Massachusetts	939	6% and over	12–16%	6–8%	5	92.0%
District of Columbia	623	4–4.9%	4–8%	0–2%	0	100.0%
Rhode Island	598	6% and over	16–19%	8–16%	3	90.7%
Louisiana	581	5–5.9%	4–8%	8–16%	1	73.2%
Michigan	527	4–4.9%	8–12%	4–6%	-2	74.6%
Pennsylvania	406	6% and over	12–16%	0–2%	4	78.7%
Illinois	388	6% and over	4–8%	2–4%	-2	88.5%
Maryland	386	6% and over	4–8%	0–2%	4	87.2%
Delaware	344	4–4.9%	8–12%	0–2%	4	83.8%
USA	*304*					
Mississippi*	219	Under 2%	0–4%	2–4%	0	49.4%
Georgia*	178	2–2.9%	0–4%	0–2%	-5	75.1%

	COVID-19 death rate per million population, May 25, 2020	% of population of French descent [French colonial ancestry][a]	Francophone Canadians % of population[a]		Urban population % of total population, 2011
Washington	143	3-3.9%	2-4%		84.1%
California*	97	5-5.9%	0-2%		95.0%
Kentucky	88	2-2.9%	2-4%		58.4%
Texas*	54	Under 2%	2-4%		84.7%
Arkansas	39	Under 2%	2-4%		56.2%
Oregon	35	3-3.9%	2-4%		81.0%
Utah	32	2-2.9%	2-4%		90.6%
Canada comparator provinces					
Quebec	497	51.3%	79.95%	-2	79.0%
Ontario	154	10.7%	2.23%	-2	85.0%
Alberta	31.3	11.0%	0.68%	0	82.0%
British Columbia	31	8.5%	0.38%	2	85.0%

US states and Canadian provinces by COVID-19 death rate per million and cultural ancestry, compared with the degree of personality (temperamental) inhibition, and degree of urbanization by state and province, May 27 2020

Note: High contact cultures exhibit lower measures of everyday physical distance [higher proximity] between strangers, acquaintances and intimates, and higher rates of physical body touching. The trait of being uninhibited means not engaging in social withdrawal, avoidance or wariness in relation to persons. Uninhibited personalities are affectively spontaneous, excitable, and display a readiness to approach unfamiliar people and objects. This is not the same as sociable personalities or the gregarious temperament of the extroverted personality. The uninhibited person is not inhibited from or fearful of touching unfamiliar objects or approaching strangers. This lack of inhibition though is associated in Rentfrow et al.'s 2013 American regional geo-psychological study with anxiety and other kinds of fear states (cf. Kagan, 95). *A relatively high rate of "friendliness" (dutiful social engagement, e.g. church fellowship) is an offset to the low uninhibited personality scores in Georgia and Mississippi (Rentfrow, Figure 2); so is the relatively significant presence of Mexican-ancestry high-contact cultures in Texas and California (Kiersz, 2018; Baxter, 1970, Table 2)

(*continued*)

Table 1.10 (continued)

Note 2: The correlation coefficient of explanatory variables to the outcome variable of COVID-19 deaths per capita in US states: Italian cultural ancestry [moderate 0.68], Italian cultural ancestry first and second [strong 0.81], French cultural ancestry [weak 0.20], uninhibited personality type [moderate 0.63], urban population [weak 0.40], all cultural ancestry variables and un-inhibition [strong 0.82]. In Canada, the correlation of the explanatory variables to the outcome variable [COVID-deaths per capita]: cultural ancestry [very strong: 0.97], language [very strong 0.96]

Sources: Andy Kiersz, Where Americans say their ancestors came from, in 17 maps, Business Insider Australia, September 10, 2018 based on Minnesota Population Centre's Integrated Public Use Microdata Series for the 2017 American Community Survey; Jeffrey M Jones, Tracking Religious Affiliation, State by State, Gallup, June 2004; David Garoogian (ed.) Ancestry & Ethnicity in America: A Comparative Guide to Over 200 Ethnic Backgrounds, 2nd edition, Grey House Publishing, 2012 based on US Census Bureau, American Community Survey, 2006–2010 Five-Year Estimates; Iowa State University, Iowa Community Indicators Program, Urban Percentage of the Population for States, Historical based on Decennial Census, U.S. Census Bureau; Statistics Canada; Canada 2011 National Household Survey; Canadian Census 2011; Cheryl Albas and Daniel Albas (1989) Aligning Actions: The Case of Subcultural Proxemics, Canadian Ethnic Studies, 21:2; Statista, Number of coronavirus (COVID-19) deaths in Canada as of May 25, 2020, by province or territory; Rentfrow, P. J. et al. (2013) Divided we stand: Three psychological regions of the United States and their political, economic, social, and health correlates. Journal of Personality and Social Psychology, 105(6), 996–1012, Fig. 2 Maps of multistate personality clusters; Jerome Kagan, Galen's Prophecy: Temperament in Human Nature, New York, Basic Books, 1994; J.C. Baxter, Interpersonal Spacing in Natural Settings. Sociometry 33 (4), pp. 444–456 (1970)

[a]Proxy for high-contact culture

[b]Ten US states have the highest percentage [6% or over] of Italian cultural ancestry, a proxy indicator of high-contact culture; eight of those states as of May 27, 2020, had higher than the national average COVID-19 deaths per capita

measure that was made famous by the American political scientist Robert Putnam: degrees of "civic" behaviour by region, that is, membership of clubs, societies, choirs and the like. To a moderately significant degree, the higher the rate of "civic" behaviour, the higher the rate of deaths per capita in Italy's regions.

As with all social phenomena, there are wheels within wheels. Take the case of Sweden. Outwardly it is a low-contact culture. Swedes are well-known for keeping their distance. "Swedes need space. A lot of space."[26] "A little more than an arm's length of personal space is common during conversations. Even when amongst family and friends, individual space is maintained. Swedish people really like to have their own personal space. For example, in elevators they tend to stand as far apart as humanly possible. Light touching is acceptable when conversing with friends and family; a hand on the arm or elbow is not uncommon."[27] So you'd expect that Sweden would do well if social proximity was a major factor in the dissemination of the virus. But Sweden's deaths per capita from COVID-19 proved to be relatively high. On the other hand you might explain that by saying that Sweden refused to lockdown its society and economy. But then you'd have to explain why countries with severe lockdowns like Britain, Italy, and Spain had a higher mortality rate per capita than Sweden did (Table 1.3). Another explanation, used even by the Swedes, is that their death rate was accounted for by the spread of the virus in their nursing homes, which they failed to effectively quarantine. The difficulty with this explanation is that, compared to the Swedes, neighbouring Norway had a still higher percentage of total COVID-related deaths in their nursing homes drawn from a much smaller national pool of nursing home residents—and yet Norway ended up with a substantially lower death rate per capita than Sweden (Table 1.1).

Then again, perhaps Sweden's operative model of social interaction is not as low-contact as might appear at first glance. Sweden's style of personal interaction is culturally quite distinct. Outwardly it is very individualistic.[28] A substantial percentage of its population live in solo households (Table 1.5). Though, contrary to reputation, no higher number than in Italy. Rather what is distinctive about Sweden is its paradoxical culture of being "alone together" (Törnqvist 2019).[29] That is, it is a society of individualized collectivists. The individualized component of the paradox is expressed in and through physical distance in interactions. The collectivist component of the paradox is expressed less through the intimate zone of personal interaction and more through what Edward Hall called personal

Table 1.11 Italy COVID-19 deaths per capita by region May 26, 2020 compared with population density and civic intensity

Region	Population January 2019	Total COVID-19 deaths by region as of April 16	Deaths per million population	Population density, persons per km²	Most civic (1) to least civic regions (9)[a]
Lombardy	10,060,574	15,896	1580	436	2
Aosta Valley	125,666	143	1138	38	4
Liguria	1,550,640	1431	923	287	2
Emilia-Romagna	4,459,477	4076	914	201	1
Piedmont	4,356,406	3812	875	173	3
Marche	1,525,271	996	653	162	3
Trentino-South Tyrol	1,072,276	461	430	87	1
Veneto	4,905,854	1866	380	282	3
Abruzzo	1,311,580	400	305	121	6
Tuscany	3,729,641	1021	274	163	1
Friuli-Venezia Giulia	1,215,220	329	271	160	2
Apulia	4,029,053	494	123	209	8
Lazio	5,879,082	693	118	347	5
Umbria	882,015	75	85	106	3
Sardinia	1,639,591	130	79	69	6
Molise	305,617	22	72	69	8
Campania	5,801,692	405	70	426	9
Sicily	4,999,891	271	54	195	7
Calabria	1,947,131	96	49	128	9
Basilicata	562,869	27	48	56	7
Italy	60,359,546	32,955	546		

Source: Statista, Coronavirus (COVID-19) deaths in Italy as of May 26, 2020, by region; Eurostat, Population density by NUTS 2 region, 2018; Robert Putnam, Making Democracy Work: Civic Traditions in Modern Italy, Princeton, Princeton University Press, 1993, Fig. 4.4, 97

Note: The correlation coefficient of explanatory variables to the outcome variable of COVID deaths per capita by region: civic behaviour [moderate 0.59], population density [weak 0.27]

[a]"Civic" refers to membership of associations, clubs, choirs, music groups, literary circles, and the like

and social zones.[30] The latter fall short of public interaction. Sweden's distinctive culture of interaction encourages forms of autonomous solidarity, independent interdependency, friendship in a domestic setting, individualists who are part of group, sociable autonomy, and forms of personal autonomy enacted together with others—along with individualist forms of collectivism, state individualism, residential sociability combined with intimate diffidence, friendly lonerism, reclusive conviviality, loose community, detached loves, companionable privacy and other kinds of social ambidexterity. This does not make for easy comparison with other nations but it does explain why in this rather unique case habitual psychological-physical distance (the sense of personal space) does not neatly translate into social distance. This is also a reminder of how heterogeneous the spread of the virus was—with sharply differing effects on neighbouring countries and regions—and how subtle micro-social factors have very visible macro-social impacts.

What applied at a national and regional level almost certainly applied also at a sub-regional level. The fractal pattern of the spread of COVID-19 went all the way down. New York State for example had high levels of COVID-related deaths in some counties but not in others.[31] I would caution against the prognosis that urban density explains this. As Tables 1.5, 1.10 and 1.11 illustrate, there is no effective explanatory correlation between urban density and per capita death rates. That is also the (reluctant) conclusion of Rader et al. (2020, April 20).[32] That study looked at the role of climate and urbanization in the spread of the disease in China. Drawing on prefecture level data it analysed the relationship of epidemic peaks to the "mean crowding" of urban density and "patchiness" of urban clustering as well as daily mean temperature and specific humidity. The study, against expectation, found that epidemic intensity was significantly negatively correlated with mean population crowding. The research did not find more epidemic intensity in crowded areas. More crowded cities experienced less intense virus outbreaks. The reason for this, the study suggested, was "crowding enables more widespread and sustained transmission between households leading incidence to be more widely distributed in time". But that speculation likely attributes to crowding in the sense of persons per square kilometre a causality that it does not possess. Close physical contact between persons—centimetres of separation, the necessary medium of COVID transmission—is not the same thing as urban population density. One can live in a dense urban setting without necessarily interacting in a physically close—"in your face"—manner. We are talking here about two different kinds of crowding—one is the number of persons per square kilometre; the other is the habitual personal space between individuals who know each other.

NOTES

1. Severe acute respiratory syndrome coronavirus 2.
2. For reasons of clarity and ease of understanding for readers who are not science professionals, I have chosen to use the abbreviation R_E rather than the more technical notation R_t for the effective reproduction rate.
3. Buitrago-Garcia, D.C. et al. (2020, April 29) analysed eight prior studies and estimated on that basis an upper bound for the proportion of asymptomatic cases to be 29%. 40–60% of all SARS-CoV-2 infections, the study estimated, were the result of transmission from pre-symptomatic individuals.
4. Statistik över antal avlidna i covid-19, April 272,020, from Sweden's National Board of Health. A Chinese study (Xie et al. 2020, April 10) of 168 patients who died in 21 hospitals in Wuhan in January 2020 concluded that "(75.0%) were men. The median (IQR) age was 70 (64–78) years, and 161 patients (95.8%) were older than 50 years… Hypertension was the most common comorbidity (84 patients [50.0%]), followed by diabetes (42 patients [25.0%]), and ischemic heart disease (31 patients [18.5%])." As of April 14, 2020, 97.4% of persons in New York City whose deaths were related to COVID-19 had an underlying condition. 60% were men (NYC Health 2020, April 14). In Italy as of April 23, 96.4% of persons who had died with COVID-19 had 1–3 comorbidities. The median age of death was 81. 63.6% were men. (SARS-CoV-2 Surveillance Group, 2020)
5. National Health Service, *COVID-19 total deaths – weekly summaries*, June 11, 2020.
6. See also The Foundation for Research on Equal Opportunity (FREOPP), Reported Deaths from COVID-19 in Long Term Care Facilities. Data used in the current work was reported by May 202,020 and tabulated in FREOPP's continuously updated spreadsheet: https://docs.google.com/spreadsheets/d/17JmyFzOd3ZEYCGpP0mK51S_Pl0yPgCuYF8PYALKuTs8/edit#gid=31142859
7. On March 29, 2020, giving evidence to the UK House of Commons Science and Technology Committee Neil Ferguson, the Imperial College London epidemiologist, put it this way: "We don't know what the level of 'excess' deaths will be, in this epidemic, by excess deaths I mean by the end of the year, what proportion of those people who died from COVID-19

would have died any-how, but it might be as much as half—half to two thirds of the deaths we are seeing from covid-19. Because it is affecting people either at the end of their lives or with poor health conditions."
8. This is what in effect what Streeck et al. 2020, April 9, recommended after their study of Gangelt in Germany: "[The already-infected] 15 percent of the population reduces the speed (net number of reproductions R in epidemiological models) of a further spread of SARS-CoV-2. By adhering to stringent hygiene measures, it can be expected that the virus concentration in the event of an infection in a person can be reduced to such an extent that the severity of the disease is reduced, while at the same time developing immunity."
9. The innate immune response of the body causes bodily "inflammation". When the immune response is uncontrolled, this can result in substantial damage to uninfected body tissue.
10. Centres for Disease Control, Disease Burden of Influenza, Figure 1: Estimated Range of Annual Burden of Flu in the U.S. since 2010.
11. Sweden, Los Angeles, Milan, Luxembourg, France, Indiana, Spain, Switzerland 1 and 2, Czech Republic, Slovenia, Sweden 1 and 2, Idaho, Madrid, Iran, Kobe, Denmark, Sweden, New York 1 and 2, International, Miami-Dade, Northern France 1 and 2, Wuhan, Chelesa Street, Santa Clara, Netherlands, Germany, Finland, Scotland, Denmark, San Francisco, San Miguel. An on-going list of these studies was tabulated by Dr. James M. Todaro at: https://docs.google.com/spreadsheets/d/1zC3kW1sMu0sjnT_vP1sh4zL0tF6fIHbA6fc-G5RQdqSc/htmlview?usp=gmail#gid=0
12. "The inferred IFR was obtained by dividing the number of deaths by the number of infected people. A corrected IFR is also presented, trying to account for the fact that only one or two types of antibodies (among IgG, IgM, IgA) might have been used." Ioannidis 2020, May 19.
13. On March 31, 2020 the biostatistician K. Wittkowski noted that the 2003 SARS virus had run its course in nations and regions for a median period of 44 days (1.4 months) and ranging from 20 days (0.6 months) to 103 days (3.4 months). For the COVID-19 virus his estimate was that it "takes at least a month from the first case entering the country (typically followed by others) for the epidemic to be detected, about three weeks for the number of cases to peak and a month for the epidemic to 'resolve'", with an incidental or zero number of cases ongoing—i.e. around three months total. Wittkowski 2020, March 31, p. 15. The current work (Table 1.3) suggests 120 days average—around four months total.
14. As Carl Heneghan and Tom Jefferson of Oxford University's Centre for Evidence-Based Medicine put it: "In the midst of a pandemic, it is easy to forget Farr's Law, and think the number infected will just keep rising, it

will not… most of all we must remember the message Farr left us: what goes up must come down." (Heneghan and Jefferson 2020, April 11)
15. An Intensive Care National Audit and Research Centre, London, study looked at 6720 critical care COVID-19 patients. The median age of admission was 62 years-old, 72% were males. Of 4078 admissions with outcomes, 2067 died [50.7%] and 2011 were discharged. Of those receiving advanced respiratory support (mechanical breathing etc.), 65% died. ICNARC 2020, April 24, Table 1 and 9.
16. There is a strong positive correlation between sunshine duration and temperature. See for example Besselaar et al. 2015.
17. "Other households" was used as a proxy for inter-generational households as the category "other households" excludes couple, single parent and sole-person households.
18. Liu et al. (2020, April 27) undertook a study of COVID-19 aerosol (airborne) transmission in the enclosed spaces of a Wuhan hospital and found little evidence of it except in crowded spaces and unventilated spaces including toilet cubicles.
19. As of April 2 the Heinsberg area—where Gangelt is located—had a population of 250,000 and a death rate from COVID-19 of 156 per million, a significant figure.
20. The reference is to after-ski-parties held in Ischgl, Austria, a scene of high-energy revelling in bars, pubs, clubs and discos.
21. The references are to a Champions League football match played in Milan on February 19, 2020 attended by 40,000 fans from nearby Bergamo and to carnival celebrations in Gangelt on February 15, 2020.
22. In the Champions League/Bergamo case, it is surmised that the virus spread was "exacerbated by the outcome of the game, as fans hugged and kissed each time Atalanta (the team from Bergamo) scored" (Avery et al. 2020, April, p. 11).
23. In a study of 3 hospitals in the Hubei region, Li et al. (2020, January 29) identified 105 COVID patients who had a recent history of travel or exposure to high-risk sites and 392 household contacts. Secondary transmission of COVID developed in 64 of the 392 household contacts (16.3%). The secondary attack rate of children was 4% compared to 17.1% for adults.
24. The reference is to the *Diamond Princess* cruise-ship and the messianic Shincheonji Church of Jesus in Daegu, South Korea, the Pentecostal Bethany Slavic Missionary church in Sacramento, California and the evangelical church of Bourtzwiller in Mulhouse, France, among others. A Singapore study examined three COVID clusters involving 28 transmitted cases. Two of the clusters originated in church congregations and one in a family gathering. Yong et al. 2020, April 21.
25. Fractal refers to a structure whose patterns recur at ever smaller scales.

26. The Swedish Toolkit book series.
27. Cultural Crossing Guide, Sweden, Personal Space & Touching, https://guide.culturecrossing.net/
28. Sweden scores 71 out of 100 for individualism on Geert Hofstede's 6-dimensions of national culture index. https://www.hofstede-insights.com/country/sweden/
29. Törnqvist's study focuses only on the small minority of Swedes who live in collective housing but the ethos of this group places in sharp relief a broader social ethos whose mentalities and mores are comparable even if the housing arrangements are different. The small group makes explicit what is implicit and buried in the habits and mentality of the broader society.
30. Hall defined the intimate zone as up to 45 centimetres; the personal as 45–140 cm; 140–365 cm.
31. Very high in the southern counties in and around New York City (such as Suffolk, Bronx, West-Chester) but very low in the northern parts of the state.
32. The study also found only weak correlation coefficients between mean temperature, mean specific humidity, population size and COVID peaks.

REFERENCES

Anon (2020, April 2). How German scientists hope to find coronavirus answers in country's worst-hit spot. *The Local*, April 2.
Arons, M.M. et al. (2020, April 24). "Presymptomatic SARS-CoV-2 Infections and Transmission in a Skilled Nursing Facility", *The New England Journal of Medicine*.
Aronson J. K. et al. (2020, April 14). 'When will it be over?': An introduction to viral reproduction numbers, R0 and Re. *Centre for Evidence Based Medicine*, Oxford University.
Avery, C. et al. (2020, April). Policy Implications of Models of the Spread of Coronavirus: Perspectives and Opportunities for Economists. *NBER Working Paper Series*, Working Paper 27007. doi:https://doi.org/10.3386/w27007
van den Besselaar, E. J. M. et al. (2015). Relationship between sunshine duration and temperature trends across Europe since the second half of the twentieth century. *Journal of Geophysical Research: Atmospheres* 120, 10,823–10,836. doi:10.1002/2015JD023640
Bi, Q. et al. (2020, April 27). Epidemiology and transmission of COVID-19 in 391 cases and 1286 of their close contacts in Shenzhen, China: a retrospective cohort study. *The Lancet Infectious Diseases*, corrected version May 5, 2020. doi:https://doi.org/10.1016/S1473-3099(20)30287-5

Buitrago-Garcia, D.C. et al. (2020, April 29). The role of asymptomatic SARS-CoV-2 infections: Rapid living systematic review and meta-analysis. *medRxiv* preprint. https://www.medrxiv.org/content/10.1101/2020.04.25.20079103v1.full.pdf

Burke, R.M. et al. (2020, March 6). Active Monitoring of Persons Exposed to Patients with Confirmed COVID-19—United States, January–February 2020. *Morbidity and Mortality Weekly Report* 69(9). US Department of Health and Human Services/Centers for Disease Control and Prevention.

Chen, Y. et al. (2020, March 4). The epidemiological characteristics of infection in close contacts of COVID-19 in Ningbo city. *Chinese Journal of Epidemiology* 41, 2020 preprint. doi:https://doi.org/10.1016/j.ijid.2020.04.034

Cheng, H-Y. et al. (2020, May 1). Contact Tracing Assessment of COVID-19 Transmission Dynamics in Taiwan and Risk at Different Exposure Periods Before and After Symptom Onset. *JAMA Internal Medicine*. https://doi.org/10.1001/jamainternmed.2020.2020

Comas-Herrera, A. et al. (2020, April 26). *Mortality associated with COVID-19 outbreaks in care homes: early international evidence.* International Long Term Care Policy Network.

Eisenberg, J. (2020, February 5). R0: How scientists quantify the intensity of an outbreak like coronavirus and predict the pandemic's spread. *The Conversation.*

Facher, L. (2020, March 11). NIH official suggests large gatherings should be canceled due to coronavirus outbreak. *STAT.*

Fauci, A.S. et al. (2020, February 26). Covid-19—Navigating the Uncharted. *The New England Journal of Medicine*, 382(13). https://doi.org/10.1056/NEJMe2002387

Ferguson, N. F. et al. (2020, March 16). *Impact of non-pharmaceutical interventions (NPIs) to reduce COVID-19 mortality and healthcare demand.* https://www.imperial.ac.uk/media/imperial-college/medicine/mrc-gida/2020-03-16-COVID19-Report-9.pdf

Ghinai, I. et al. (2020, March 13). First known person-to-person transmission of severe acute respiratory syndrome coronavirus 2 (SARS-CoV-2) in the USA. *The Lancet* 395 (10230), 1137–1144. doi:https://doi.org/10.1016/S0140-6736(20)30607-3

Girvan, G. & Roy, A. (2020, May 8 updated May 22). Nursing Homes & Assisted Living Facilities Account for 42% of COVID-19 Deaths. *FREOPP.*

Hall, E. T. (1966). *The Hidden Dimension.* Garden City, N.Y.: Doubleday.

Heneghan, C. & Jefferson, T. (2020, April 11). COVID-19: William Farr's way out of the Pandemic. *Centre for Evidence-Based Medicine.*

ICNAR Intensive Care National Audit & Research Centre. (2020, April 24). *ICNARC report on COVID-19 in critical care.*

1 SOCIAL DISTANCE   37

Ioannidis, J. (2020, May 19). The infection fatality rate of COVID-19 inferred from seroprevalence data. *medRxiv* preprint. Updated July 14. doi:https://doi.org/10.1101/2020.05.13.20101253

Jing, Q-L. et al. (2020, April 15). Household Secondary Attack Rate of COVID-19 and Associated Determinants. *medRxiv* preprint. doi:https://doi.org/10.1101/2020.04.11.20056010

Li, Q. et al. (2020, January 29). Early Transmission Dynamics in Wuhan, China, of Novel Coronavirus–Infected Pneumonia. *The New England Journal of Medicine*. doi:https://doi.org/10.1056/NEJMoa2001316

Liu, Y. et al. (2020, April 27). Aerodynamic analysis of SARS-CoV-2 in two Wuhan hospitals. *Nature*. https://www.nature.com/articles/s41586-020-2271-3

NYC Health. (2020, April 14). *Coronavirus Disease 2019 (COVID-19) Daily Data Summary*.

Phaneuf, K. M. (2020, April 20). COVID-19 caused more deaths among CT nursing home residents than initially reported. *The CT Mirror*.

Qian, H. et al. (2020, April 7). Indoor transmission of SARS-CoV-2. *medRxiv* preprint. doi:https://doi.org/10.1101/2020.04.04.20053058

Rader, B. et al. (2020, April 20). Crowding and the epidemic intensity of 1 COVID-19 transmission. *medRxiv* preprint. https://doi.org/10.1101/2020.04.15.20064980

SARS-CoV-2 Surveillance Group. (2020). Characteristics of SARS-CoV-2 patients dying in Italy Report based on available data on April 23th, 2020. Istituto Superiore Sanità.

Sekine, T. et al. (2020, June 29) Robust T cell immunity in convalescent individuals with asymptomatic or mild COVID-19. bioRxiv preprint. https://doi.org/10.1101/2020.06.29.174888

Streeck, H. et al. (2020, April 9). *Vorläufiges Ergebnis und Schlussfolgerungen der COVID-19 Case-ClusterStudy (Gemeinde Gangelt)*. https://www.land.nrw/sites/default/files/asset/document/zwischenergebnis_covid19_case_study_gangelt_0.pdf

Swan, N. (2020, April 13). Interview with Professor Ian Frazer, Faculty of Medicine, University of Queensland. *Health Report*. Australian Broadcasting Corporation.

Törnqvist, M. (2019). Living Alone Together: Individualized Collectivism in Swedish Communal Housing. *Sociology* 53(5), 900–915.

Wingerter, M. (2020, April 22). Residents of nursing homes, assisted living facilities now account for 64% of Colorado's coronavirus deaths. *Denver Post*.

Wittkowski, K.M. (2020, March 31). The first three months of the COVID-19 epidemic: Epidemiological evidence for two separate strains of SARS-CoV-2 viruses spreading and implications for prevention strategies. *medRxiv* preprint. doi:https://doi.org/10.1101/2020.03.28.20036715

Xie, J., et al. (2020, April 10). Clinical Characteristics of Patients Who Died of Coronavirus Disease 2019 in China. *Research Letter, Critical Care Medicine,* JAMA Network Open. https://doi.org/10.1001/jamanetworkopen.2020.5619

Yong, S.E.F. et al. (2020, April 21). Connecting clusters of COVID-19: an epidemiological and serological investigation. *The Lancet Infectious Diseases.* doi:https://doi.org/10.1016/S1473-3099(20)30273-5

Zhu, Y., et al. (2020, March 30). Children are unlikely to have been the primary source of household SARS-CoV-2 infections. *medRxiv* preprint. doi:https://doi.org/10.1101/2020.03.26.20044826

CHAPTER 2

Public Policy

Abstract The chapter examines various public policy measures in response to COVID-19 from advisories, testing and tracking through to lockdowns of economy and society. The role of epidemiological modelling in making public policy, proportionality in decision-making, the weighing of competing goods, and the unintended consequences of public policy decisions are discussed.

Keywords Competing goods • Control • Distance • Economic costs • Social costs • Households • Government • Public policy • Hospitals • Humility • Intervention • Judgment • Prudence • Life span • Middle way • Mitigation • Suppression • Modelling • Residential care homes • Observation • Pattern • Planning • Pluralism • Proportionality • Public opinion • Restrictions • Targeting • Uncertainty • Unintended consequences

March and April 2020 saw a dramatic development in public policy across most of the world. In March, governments began to sponsor social distancing policies—first by advising populations to physically distance and then implementing regimes to test persons who might be infected, track their contacts and quarantine confirmed carriers of the virus at home (Table 2.1). A range of prohibitions short of comprehensive social shutdown were also progressively introduced (Table 2.2). This was followed in

Table 2.1 Number of COVID-19 tests per million by country and date

Country	COVID-19-related deaths per million pop, April 26,2020	January 21	February 1	February 15	March 1	March 15	April 1
Spain	580						175
United Kingdom	546		3	44	175	598	2272
Italy	545				0	357	9156
France	437				37	559	3412
Sweden	408				109	1423	3656
Netherlands	342					939	4533
United States	304				0	79	3473
Switzerland	221						15,074
Canada	176					1435	6833
Germany	101				1064	2609	11,205
Denmark	97					1851	4677
Hungary	52					955	
Norway	43					3314	17,297
Japan	7			8	20	103	273
South Korea	5	0	7	146	1883	5207	8184
Australia	4					5633	10,276
Singapore	4						11,111
Hong Kong	0.5						12,911
Taiwan	0.3					723	1416

Source: OurWorldinData, COVID-19 confirmed deaths versus tests, https://ourworldindata.org/grapher/covid-19-tests-deaths-scatter-with-comparisons; Hong Kong Department of Health, Data in Coronavirus Disease (COVID-19) https://data.gov.hk/en-data/dataset/hk-dh-chpsebcddr-novel-infectious-agent; Singapore Ministry of Health, Number of Covid-19 Tests Performed and Daily Updates On National Health Statistics for Comparison, April 6 2020 https://www.moh.gov.sg/news-highlights/details/number-of-covid-19-tests-performed-and-daily-updates-on-national-health-statistics-for-comparison

Note: if data for nominated date is not available, data for the closest date is used. Sweden April 1 figure is from March 29; Denmark March 15 figure is from March 20; Germany March 1 figure is March 8; Germany April 1 figure is March 29; Norway March 15 figure is March 16; Canada March 15 figure is March 18; Australia March 15 figure is March 22; Australia April 1 figure is April 2; Japan February 15 figure is February 14; Taiwan March 15 figure is March 21; Singapore April 1 figure is April 6

Table 2.2 Early COVID-19 mitigation actions taken December–March 2020

Date of actions undertaken	Australia	Canada	Denmark	France	Germany	Hong Kong	Italy	Japan	Netherlands	Norway	Singapore	South Korea	Spain	Sweden	Switzerland	Taiwan	UK	USA
Last week Dec						FS												
First week Jan											FS					FS		TA
Second week Jan																		TA
Third week Jan																ME		
Fourth+ week Jan		TA FB EX				SE SC TB SPC	SE TB				HQ NHR BC						TA	
First week Feb	TA HQ BC	EX			EX			TB CSQ EX			HQ	TB TA				TB HQ SC	HQ	AQ
Second week Feb																TA	HQ	
Third week Feb											TR GEP			TA				EX
Fourth+ week Feb			HQ	LGB	HQ FS		MDL	SC SPC HQ	TA		TA	IZ	TA		LGB	TB GEP TR	TA	SCI TA TB
First week March	TC SPC	TA	TR HQ NHR	SCP SPC	ME	EX	SC SPC	TA	TA		TB HQ	SC HBI GEP		T A TB	SC BC LGB			SCI

Second week March	LGB GEP	TB SE[a] SC MDLD	SD MLD LGB BC	LGB	SC MLD SPC GB GEP NHR	SLD	LGB FB BC	SC SPC NHR SD TR TA NHR FB GEP	NHR	IZ	SE MDL GEP FB BC LGB	LGB	SLD GEP LGB	HQ TA	TB
Third week March	HQ BC SD MDL	SE[a] SC MDL	SD BC SC GB	SD	SE MDL GB TB	TB HQ HOQ MLD	SD SC SPC MDL GEP NHR					SD SPC			TB TR	ME SC LGB SPC	StLDs
Fourth+ week March	GB MDL SCP GEP	GEP TB	SLD	SLD	MDL GEP MD							LGB TSO			SLD	StLDs

Abbreviations: AQ Airport quarantine centres, BC Border closure, CSQ Cruise Ship Quarantine, EX Extraction of citizens, FB Flight ban, FS Flight screening, GB Gatherings banned, GEP Government economic package, HBI Hospital beds increased, HOQ Hotel quarantine, HQ Home quarantine, IZ Isolation zones mandated, LGB Large gatherings banned, MDL Moderate lockdown, ME Medical equipment masks, MLD Mild lockdown, NEH Non-essential hospital operations restricted, NHR Nursing home restrictions, SC Schools closed, SCI School closure incidental, SCP School closure partial, SD Formal social distancing rules, SE State of emergency declared, SLD Severe lockdown, StLD State lockdowns, SPC Sports cancelled, TA Travel advisory, TR Traveller restrictions, TSO Table service only [restaurants]

[a]States

April 2020 by governments locking down their economies (to varying degrees) to further reduce physical interaction between people. Tables 2.3 and 2.4 indicate the relative intensity of these shutdowns by nation.

In the absence of government prohibitions, four factors in principle could reduce the reproduction number of COVID-19: a vaccine, community immunity, social distancing and environmental conditions. In addition, re-purposing an existing drug might provide an effective therapy for persons in critical care. There was little chance of a vaccine being developed early enough to combat the virus spread in 2020. In March–April 2020, drug therapy was also uncertain. A public policy argument that was common in the latter part of March 2020 boiled down to the following: community immunity will reduce the R_0 number in the long run. But in the interim, if the R_0 number is high or very high, the resulting influx of

Table 2.3 Workplace location visits and length of stay against a baseline of Jan 3–Feb 6, 2020 activity

Country	March 23–29	March 30–April 5	April 6–12	April 13–19	April 20–26	May 4–10	May 11–17
Spain	-66%	-72%	-75%	-67%	-64%	-55%	-49%
United Kingdom	-58%	-65%	-67%	-66%	-61%	-60%	-55%
Italy	-68%	-67%	-66%	-65%	-61%	-42%	-38%
France	-68%	-67%	-65%	-66%	-60%	-55%	-37%
Sweden	-24%	-26%	-40%	-33%	-21%	-19%	-19%
Netherlands	-45%	-44%	-43%	-45%	-38%	-36%	-28%
United States	-42%	-46%	-49%	-45%	-44%	-39%	-37%
Switzerland	-47%	-46%	-51%	-49%	-40%	-30%	-23%
Canada	-53%	-56%	-60%	-55%	-52%	-47%	-45%
Germany	-41%	-39%	-46%	-43%	-30%	-9%	-8%
Denmark	-47%	-45%	-55%	-43%	-32%	-29%	-24%
Hungary	-42%	-42%	-50%	-46%	-37%	-30%	-29%
Norway	-46%	-44%	-60%	-44%	-35%	-28%	-22%
Japan	-5%	-10%	-17%	-22%	-25%	-45%	-22%
South Korea	-7%	-7%	-6%	-11%	-3%	-12%	-2%
Australia	-23%	-33%	-45%	-43%	-36%	-31%	-29%
Singapore	-13%	-17%	-55%	-60%	-63%	-63%	-62%
Hong Kong	-17%	-25%	-23%	-28%	-16%	-9%	-8%
Taiwan	-13%	-16%	4%	4%	4%	4%	3%

Source: Google COVID-19 Global Mobility Report May 27 2020

Note: The baseline is the median value, for the corresponding day of the week, during the 5-week period Jan 3–Feb 6, 2020

Table 2.4 Retail and recreation location visits and length of stay against a baseline of Jan 3–Feb 6, 2020 activity

Country	March 23–29	March 30–April 5	April 6–12	April 13–19	April 20–26	May 4–10	May 11–17
Spain	-88%	-91%	-91%	-89%	-88%	-78%	-71%
United Kingdom	-72%	-76%	-76%	-75%	-73%	-72%	-69%
Italy	-84%	-88%	-84%	-84%	-82%	-62%	-59%
France	-84%	-87%	-83%	-83%	-80%	-74%	-49%
Sweden	-22%	-24%	-22%	-22%	-13%	-15%	-17%
Netherlands	-48%	-46%	-44%	-45%	-36%	-31%	-31%
United States	-42%	-42%	-45%	-41%	-39%	-29%	-28%
Switzerland	-71%	-80%	-76%	-75%	-71%	-56%	-35%
Canada	-53%	-55%	-56%	-53%	-55%	-42%	-40%
Germany	-62%	-55%	-52%	-57%	-49%	-37%	-32%
Denmark	-37%	-31%	-29%	-28%	-20%	-24%	-21%
Hungary	-56%	-53%	-52%	-53%	-47%	-31%	-30%
Norway	-46%	-40%	-43%	-37%	-25%	-17%	-12%
Japan	-8%	-14%	-23%	-33%	-37%	-32%	-32%
South Korea	-19%	-16%	-15%	-13%	-13%	-2%	-6%
Australia	-31%	-41%	-44%	-40%	-39%	-29%	-26%
Singapore	-19%	-22%	-52%	-61%	-67%	-65%	-63%
Hong Kong	-28%	-31%	-24%	-28%	-25%	-18%	-18%
Taiwan	7%	-11%	-14%	-10%	-16%	-8%	-9%

Source: Google Global Mobility Report May 27 2020

Note: The baseline is the median value, for the corresponding day of the week, during the 5-week period Jan 3–Feb 6, 2020

serious and critical cases could put undue pressure on a nation's hospital system. In lieu of a vaccine or an effective therapy, and a R_0 number between 2 and 3, this left governments with a third mitigating factor: human agency. In short, the ability to distance oneself from others.

A series of public health measures were introduced in March 2020—social distancing advisories, advice to regularly and thoroughly wash hands and clean surfaces regularly touched, travel advisories, travel restrictions, flight screening, testing and tracing infected persons, home quarantining of infected persons, flight bans, nursing home restrictions, temporary school closures, border closures, sports cancellations, bans on gatherings and the hotel quarantining of infected persons. These were largely—though not entirely—proportionate to a serious health issue. The best of these measures addressed key characteristics of the virus spread. Social distancing targeted the specific nature of the transmission of the disease that occurs through close physical contact—especially within families and between relatives and friends. Tracking and tracing targeted persons who were ill from the virus or who had contracted it (Tables 2.1 and 2.2). Nursing home advisories and restrictions targeted persons in nursing homes who were at particular risk of dying from the disease or with the disease present in their autopsies.

Other aspects of the March 2020 public policy phalanx appeared excessive. Closing schools to prevent the spread of the virus among the very low-risk population of children and their young adult parents was an example.[1] In the state of New South Wales in Australia, from March to mid-April 2020 there were 18 cases of students with the virus out of a total school population of 1.1 million (NCIRS 2020). 735 students and 128 staff had close contacts with the 18 cases. No teacher or staff member contracted the virus from any of the cases. One primary school and one high school child may have contracted COVID-19 from the 18 carriers. Even within households, it was adults not children who were the primary transmission agents of the virus (Zhu et al. 2020, March 30). Death from the virus among children was negligible—unlike many of the more virulent seasonal flus.

Despite this, governments and public health authorities in many jurisdictions insisted on closing schools. The reason why is evident from a reporter's exchange with Jeannette Young Queensland's Chief Health Officer (CHO) and Australia's longest serving CHO (Lynch 2020). Young explained why she told the Premier of Queensland to shut down schools on March 26 even though evidence showed that schools were not a high-risk environment for the spread of the virus.[2] The "reason" was that closing schools down would help people understand the gravity of the situation. In other words it was to scare people. The measure had no rational basis. This came from a senior health official who, after the first case in Queensland was confirmed on January 25, concluded that this "is going to be a nightmare". "[My] advice to the Premier was, 'we have to throw everything at this'." But how much was this a self-fulfilling prophecy? And one with very little evidence to support it.[3]

On February 24 the World Health Organization (WHO) published a report on China, the original source of the virus outbreak. The WHO report concluded several pertinent facts: the primary route of transmission was via households, there was a relatively low attack rate for individuals aged 18 years old and under, transmission in hospitals and health-care settings was relatively rare, there were reports of transmission in closed settings involving close proximity such as prisons and a long-term care facility, and the susceptibility to the virus skewed towards much older persons (the WHO estimated a mean age of 51, which later would be raised substantially).[4] "Within Wuhan," the WHO reported, "among testing of ILI samples, no children were positive in November and December of 2019 and in the first two weeks of January 2020" (WHO 2020, p. 11). Individuals, the WHO observed, who were at highest risk of severe disease and death were persons aged over 60 and those with underlying conditions such as hypertension, diabetes, cardiovascular disease, chronic respiratory disease and cancer (WHO 2020, p. 12). That was a pretty accurate profile of who was most susceptible to the virus. In spite of that, governments and public health officials proceeded to shut down schools.

Worse still was the story of those in nursing homes. Nursing home residents were the population most at risk from COVID-19. They were old, often with multiple comorbidities, and living in large numbers in close proximity in an enclosed space. It is an obvious and much more efficient strategy to quarantine the most at risk rather than the least at risk or whole populations. Not only did this not happen but (to the contrary) hospitals in New York City and in the United Kingdom—locations that were among the most intensely affected by the virus—till late April decanted COVID patients from hospitals into nursing homes without requiring a test to determine the patients were no longer infectious. This decanting policy was a sign that the health system as a whole had a distorted understanding—or perhaps, more accurately, interpretation—of COVID's pattern behaviour. It was also a sign that "protecting hospital systems" from being overburdened by COVID patients was de facto a higher priority than protecting populations that were highly susceptible to the virus. This is a strong indicator that institutional priorities and anxieties were driving government and public health responses to COVID-19 rather than a grounded, evidence-based assessment of the risks and behaviour of the virus.

In mid-March Britain's National Health Service (NHS) decided to "transfer 15,000 patients out of hospitals and back into the community, including an unspecified number of patients to care homes… [These] included some who had tested positive for COVID-19, but were judged better cared for outside hospital" (Grey and Macaskill 2020). A UK Department of Health guidance note dated April 2 stated that "negative tests are not required prior to transfers/admissions into the care home."

Consequently asymptomatic and symptomatic COVID-19 patients were discharged from hospitals into care homes (Booth 2020, May 20). New York State similarly on March 26 mandated nursing homes to take COVID patients who had been discharged from hospital. The state did not reverse that mandate till May 10 (Mathews 2020a, b, March 26 & May 14). The Society for Post-Acute and Long-Term Care Medicine in March warned New York that "admitting patients with suspected or documented Covid-19 infection" represented "a clear and present danger to all of the residents of a nursing home". Michigan in the United States had a policy similar to New York's. Michigan mandated nursing homes to accept patients infected with COVID-19. As late as May 13 the state governor renewed the mandate and without releasing nursing home death statistics.

Why the peculiar emphasis on "protecting hospitals"? If we think of hospitals and public health systems as a collective ego, what we saw on display in the COVID episode was an ego that is both fragile (in need of protection) and self-important (making its own protection a greater priority than that of the most vulnerable population). The anxieties of this fragile yet vain ego were compressed in a series of vastly exaggerated modelling projections of beds required for COVID patients. What was presumed was that some kind of crisis faced hospitals that would be critically short of beds and overwhelmed by demand. What actually happened? In New York City, barely over 1000 persons were treated in a 2500-bed emergency military hospital that was constructed at the Javits Convention Center. A US navy hospital ship (Comfort) was sent to New York to support its presumed hospital bed emergency. The navy ship treated fewer than 200 patients. In the UK in the middle of April British hospitals had four times the normal number of *empty* beds (West 2020). So effective was the UK government panic about COVID bed numbers that 40.9% of NHS general acute beds were unoccupied as of April 11 and 12—37,500 out of a total of 91,600—because of ramped up discharges and directives for non-COVID patients to leave hospital. A temporary 4000-bed overflow Nightingale Hospital was built in 10 days at the ExCel conference centre at Docklands in East London. Just 54 patients were treated at the temporary facility (Campbell and Mason 2020, May 4).

In May 2020, the chair of the British Parliament's Health and Social Care Committee (HSCC), Jeremy Hunt, estimated that 20,000 of Britain's 36,000 plus deaths—55%—occurred in nursing homes.[5] This compared then with Australia's 25%, Singapore's 11% and Hong Kong's 0% (Table 1.1). Giving evidence to the HSCC, Hong Kong University's Professor Terry Lum observed that, of all possible measures, what is "most important is stopping the transmission from hospital to nursing home" (Booth 2020, May 20). To achieve this, anyone in a Hong Kong nursing home who was infected was isolated in hospital for three months. Close contacts were quarantined for two weeks for observation. Hong Kong nursing homes have trained infection controllers who regularly practice emergency drills. The most effective infection control aimed at COVID-19 was ensuring no close contact with aged relatives. Yet there are powerful built-in social expectations that militate against this. When the New South Wales government in Australia eased restrictions on family visits as a first step in relaxing its compulsory lockdown in early May 2020, the state's Health Minister articulated the ambivalence: "It's really tough to not be able to hug your mum or kiss your mum, but it would be the wisest course to not do that" (Clun 2020, May 9). The minister, in a nutshell, summed up the tension between prudent distance and the communitarian brain that is drawn to a high-touch society. Anxiety about viruses drive people apart physically—they step back from any real or imagined corporeal threat. Yet that same anxiety drives people closer together seeking physical comfort, consolation and reassurance in a period of heightened nervousness.

2.1 Proportionality

A lack of proportionate, targeted, fine-tuned and mid-range responses dogged COVID-19 public policy through March and April 2020. It is as though no public language or civic rhetoric existed anymore to deal with mid-range public matters that fall between the extremes of unimportance and catastrophe. The medium, middle and intermediate fell out of focus while the rhetoric of emergency, crisis and disaster heated up.

This is typified on a national scale by the United States which swung from doing little in March to shutdowns mostly beginning in April (Tables 2.1 and 2.2). Within a few weeks the country careened from the President calling the virus a hoax to shutdowns of variable lengths in most American states with much of the population directed to stay-at-home. In numerous countries, March restrictions on gatherings addressed the propensity of the virus to propagate in crowded enclosed spaces. But like many of the later April lockdown measures the bans on gatherings lacked finesse. These did not distinguish between enclosed and unclosed spaces, outdoor or indoor spaces, ventilated or unventilated spaces, packed or dispersed bodies, or take into account the length of time (prolonged or short) that a person might spend in an enclosed space, or identify the difference between a crowded indoor space and one that was not crowded. The lockdown measures in late March and April exhibited even less proportion and finesse. These were of a wholesale and largely undifferentiated nature. They required the closure of arbitrarily-defined "non-essential" businesses, the quarantining of whole nations and their healthy populations in their own homes, and the extended closure of schools.

In one way or another all the measures in March and April 2020 were (or rather tried to be) an artificial amplification of the habits of social distancing and inter-personal spacing that nations and regions already practiced. Governments in effect attempted to augment, magnify and intensify habitual social spacing. Did it work? Judged at least by the outcome (though the causality is unclear) the March 2020 government advisories, tracking, tracing and quarantining regimes, and targeted prohibitions (such as travel bans) had a measurable influence on the spread of the virus. German epidemiologists reported a drop in Germany's reproduction number from a high of 3.1 on March 9 2020 to an admirable low of 1 by March 21. After that, through to April 9, the reproduction number fluctuated between 0.9 and 1—a success reflected in Germany's modest death rate per capita (Table 2.5).

The results of the April 2020 measures—the lockdowns—by governments are less impressive. Germany reached the propitious reproduction number of 1 *before* its lockdown began. Death rates per capita in countries with severe lockdowns, like the United Kingdom, commonly peaked in April and then dropped—outwardly a success of the lockdown policy. But deaths per capita is a lagging indicator of infections that begin (conservatively) three weeks prior to death on average.[6] In many countries including the United Kingdom the rate of inflection (as indicated by the subsequent rate of daily deaths) had peaked and had been falling *before* the imposition of a lockdown (Table 2.6).

Given the stages of incubation followed by infection through to death or hospital discharge in serious COVID cases, any positive effect of a lockdown on the rate of death would only show itself three weeks *after* the lockdown had begun. Conversely if COVID-19 followed the characteristic symmetrical bell-curve trajectory of viruses that William Farr observed in 1840, it was predictable that the time lapse between the lip of the bell curve in its early phase to the lip of the curve in its fading days would be several months only. Japan's Ministry of Health on March 9, 2020 predicted that the COVID peak of each Japanese prefecture would occur

Table 2.5 Germany, effective reproduction number of COVID-19 compared with government actions taken

Date	Reproduction number	Government action in corresponding week
Last week of February		Home quarantines, flight monitoring
March 6	2.3	
March 9	3.1	
March 11 peak	3.3	Sports cancelled, school closures, mild lockdown measures, gatherings ban, nursing home restrictions
March 16	2.7	Moderate lockdown measures, gatherings banned, travel ban, home quarantine, hotel quarantines
March 21	1	Formal social distancing rules
March 23	0.9	Severe lockdown measures
March 26	1	
March 30	0.9	
April 1	1	
April 6	0.9	
April 9	0.9	

Source: Schätzung der aktuellen Entwicklung der SARS-CoV-2-Epidemie in Deutschland – Nowcasting, Epidemiologisches Bulletin 17, 15 April 2020, Fig. 4

"roughly three months" after their first reported case of local transmission.[7] At the end of May 2020 it looked like two months would be the average around the world (Table 1.3).

What the bell curve pattern should remind us is that nature has its own regularities—and human intervention is limited in the degree to which it can alter or reverse these. Humanity can adapt to nature's constancies (social distancing being an example) and it can re-purpose natural phenomena for its own ends (vaccines being an example). But "the government must do something to fix this now" styles of intervention rarely work effectively. They lack the modesty of successful human adaptation. Humility is a virtue too often absent from public policy.

Public and government attitudes in March 2020 and early April 2020 were strongly influenced by predictions made by researchers modelling the reproduction number of COVID-19 and what was inferred from that: the anticipated rate of death per capita and projected demand for hospital beds. Given different assumptions, the projections of deaths differed widely (Table 2.7) even within the same model. Modellers often made no clear distinction between the effective reproduction number R_E and the

Table 2.6 COVID-19 infection peak compared to lockdown timing

Nation	Date lockdown began	Daily deaths peak	Infection peak[a]	Infection peak before (B), after (A) or same (S) as lockdown start	Number of days that infection peak occurred after lockdown
Australia	March 29	April 6	March 16	B	0
Italy	March 7–9	March 27	March 6	S	0
Spain	March 28	April 2	March 12	B	0
United Kingdom	March 23	April 8[b]	March 10	B[b]	0
Austria	March 16	April 8	March 18	A	2
Germany	March 23	April 8	March 18	B	0
Denmark	March 13	April 4	March 14	S	0
France	March 16	April 15	March 25	A	9
United States	March 19–April 7	April 21	March 31	B/A	0–12
Thailand	March 26	April 3	March 13	B	0
Switzerland	March 16	April 4	March 14	B	0
Netherlands	March 15	April 7	March 17	A	2
Israel	March 19	April 2	March 12	B	0
Ireland	March 28	April 24	April 3	A	6
Finland	March 18	April 21	March 31	A	13
Croatia	March 22	April 19	March 29	A	7
New Zealand	March 26	March 28	March 7	B	0
Slovenia	March 20	April 7	March 17	B	0
Philippines	March 15	April 12	March 22	A	7
Malaysia	March 18	March 26	March 5	B	0
Lithuania	March 12	April 10	March 20	A	8

Source: Worldometer, Coronavirus, Daily deaths by nation; UK NHS COVID-19 daily deaths summary May 3 2020
[a]The infection peak is imputed. It back-dates infections three weeks prior to deaths
[b]On UK National Health Service (NHS) figures the peak occurred on April 8; April 21 is the peak according to UK Government figures, coronavirus.data.gov.uk, Coronavirus (COVID-19) in the UK

basic reproduction number R_0 of the virus. Insistent claims were made during March of 2020 that comprehensive lockdowns of the economy and society were needed to save hospital systems. The lockdown strategy was developed by Communist China. Yet most democratic nations embraced it in March.

Hospitals are flexible enough to deal with known contingencies. It is a known contingency that influenza is a recurring seasonal phenomenon

Table 2.7 Early models of the COVID-19 infection fatality rate (IFR) and projected resulting deaths assuming 60% of the population is infected

Nations, Population, Herd Immunity Threshold Population Number		Number of deaths if 60% of the population [early conjectured 'herd immunity' threshold estimate] has been infected, by the infection fatality rate (IFR) of different epidemiological models, 2020							
		CEBM[a] estimated LFR range, 0.1–0.36%							
	Population, 2019	60% of population infected ['herd immunity' threshold]	COVID-19 infection fatality rate 0.36% [highest], CEBM 17 April 2020	COVID-19 infection fatality rate 0.1% [low], CEBM 17 April 2020	COVID-19 infection fatality rate 0.5%, Timothy Russell LSHTM estimate 9 March 2020	COVID-19 infection fatality rate 0.9%, Imperial College estimate 16 March 2020	COVID-19 Wuhan infection fatality rate 0.66%, Imperial College estimate 13 March 2020	COVID-19 Diamond Princess infection fatality rate 2.9%, Imperial College estimate 13 March 2020	COVID-19 infection fatality rate 1.2%, Diamond Princess actual Nature 26 March	COVID-19 infection fatality rate various by country [0.042%–0.232%] P. Simon 10 April 2020[b]
Australia	25,203,000	15,121,800	54,438	15,122	75,609	136,096	99,804	438,532	181,462	6351
Canada	37,590,000	22,554,000	81,194	22,554	112,770	202,986	148,856	654,066	270,648	20,524
Denmark	5,806,000	3,483,600	12,541	3484	17,418	31,352	22,992	101,024	41,803	4877
Germany	83,020,000	49,812,000	179,323	49,812	249,060	448,308	328,759	1,444,548	597,744	50,310
Japan	126,860,000	76,116,000	274,018	76,116	380,580	685,044	502,366	2,207,364	913,392	46,431
Norway	5,515,000	3,309,000	11,912	3309	16,545	29,781	21,839	95,961	39,708	2250
South Korea	51,225,000	30,735,000	110,646	30,735	153,675	276,615	202,851	891,315	368,820	20,592
Switzerland	8,570,000	5,142,000	18,511	5142	25,710	46,278	33,937	149,118	61,704	11,929

Sources: Lourenço, J. et al. (2020, March 26) Fundamental principles of epidemic spread highlight the immediate need for large-scale serological surveys to assess the stage of the SARS CoV-2 epidemic, medRxiv pre-print; Simon, P. (2020, April 10) Robust Estimation of Infection Fatality Rates during the Early Phase of a Pandemic, medRxiv preprint; Ferguson, N.M. et al. (2020, March 16) Impact of non-pharmaceutical interventions (NPIs) to reduce COVID-19 mortality and healthcare demand; Russell, T.W. (2020, March 9) Estimating the infection and case fatality ratio for COVID-19 using age-adjusted data from the outbreak on the Diamond Princess cruise ship, medRxiv pre-print; Verity, R. et al. (2020, March 13) Estimates of the severity of COVID-19 disease, medRxiv preprint

Note: The infection fatality rate of seasonal flu strains is around 0.1% https://www.cdc.gov/flu/about/burden/index.html

[a]Centre for Evidence Based Medicine, Oxford University. [b]Simon's predicted IFR by country: Australia 0.042%, Canada 0.091%, Denmark 0.14%, Germany 0.101%, Japan 0.061%, Norway 0.068%, South Korea 0.067%, Switzerland 0.232%

and that there will be bad flu seasons, so hospitals ask surgeons to defer elective operations while they deal with the variable load from influenza cases year to year. However the same institutional and procedural flexibility is markedly less apparent in the case of unknown contingencies. In March 2020 the anxieties of the health modellers and planners focused on hospitals: could hospitals cope with a novel virus? The modellers and planners assumed relative inflexibility in the face of a contingency (a new virus) whose behaviour was unfamiliar. The new phenomenon could not be readily analogized with prior examples and patterns or perhaps the modelling mind lacked a sufficient range of analogies and analogical techniques to deal with novelty. Whatever the case, the modellers and health planners assumed on the part of hospitals an inability to rapidly convert ward beds to ICUs or delay elective operations in favour of urgent cases as demand required. In other words the planning and procedural mind could not imagine hospitals matching demand with supply in a flexible self-organizing manner rather than on a rigid inert basis that somehow inexorably would result in the swamping of the health system if society was not shutdown.

As March progressed, COVID hawkishness rose. It was increasingly argued that severe measures had to be imposed—in particular, the quarantining of a large portion of the healthy populations of nations. Without this, hospital systems would collapse under the weight of an over-whelming demand for beds to treat serious and critical COVID-related cases. In some cases there were apocalyptic-scale predictions of the need for hospital beds. In the end though actual demand fell markedly, often dramatically, short of the predictions (Tables 2.8 and 2.9). This is a stark reminder that modelling is not an observation of what has happened. It is a prediction of future events based on the assumptions of the modellers. Those assumptions in themselves can be more or less realistic. The probability that a successful model of the behaviour of a novel virus can be created in the early stages of the spread of a virus is low if basic behavioural attributes are not known like what percentage of the infected population will be asymptomatic or what percentage of the population have an adaptive immune response that is cross-reactive from their experience of comparable viruses. Models have to be constructed on data about past events. Yet when faced with modelling a novel event, the question remains: what bits of the past are comparable and which are not? Without extensive empirical evidence about the novel entity, this question cannot be meaningfully answered. Even then models rarely effectively model countervailing forces—be they natural or social—that can reverse a predicted course of

2 PUBLIC POLICY   55

Table 2.8   Australia, ICU and ward beds for COVID-19 peak, predicted and actual

Number of serious + critical [hospitalisation] COVID-19 cases, Australia	
February 15 (0) March 1 (0) April 1 (50) April 15 (76) April 20 (49)	
Total [baseline] hospital beds, 2017–2018	
97,500	
Predicted need for hospital ICU and ward beds for admissions [Doherty Institute, University of Melbourne]	
Scenarios assume cancellation of non-urgent surgery and reduction in admissions for conditions such as respiratory infections and traffic accidents	
Scenario A [5xbasline ICU bed capacity]	
Total ICU and ward beds for admissions during COVID-19 pandemic, worst-case scenario A	26,870
COVID ICU and ward beds for admissions [50% of total] worse-case scenario A	13,435
Scenario B [3xbasline ICU bed capacity]	
Total ICU and ward beds for admissions during COVID-19 pandemic, scenario B	16,122
COVID ICU and ward beds for admissions [50% of total] scenario B	8061
Scenario C [2xbasline ICU bed capacity]	
Total ICU and ward beds for admissions during COVID-19 pandemic, scenario C	10,748
COVID ICU and ward beds for admissions [50% of total] scenario C	5374

Sources: Australian Institute of Health and Welfare, Hospital resources 2017-18: Australian hospital statistics; Worldometer, Coronavirus data archived by date at the Internet Archive; Moss R, Wood J, Brown D, Shearer F, Black, AJ, Cheng AC, McCaw JM, McVernon J, Modelling the impact of COVID-19 in Australia to inform transmission reducing measures and health system preparedness, The Peter Doherty Institute for Infection and Immunity, The University of Melbourne and Royal Melbourne Hospital

events. This is especially true in the case of natural or social causation that is dependent on the interaction of multiple causal factors.

Modelling commonly provides a range of possible outcomes based on a range of assumptions. Some of these assumptions will be more probable or realistic than others. Many will be stabs in the dark, and not very reliable. The difficulty is that figures at the upper end of the range—the least probable ones—tend to get widely quoted because of their melodramatic character. The most exaggerated figures—all of them based on assumptions, not on empirical realities—enter the public imagination. In March and early April 2020 this kind of histrionic translation occurred on a mass scale—initially via journalists, academics, health officials and government ministers. What followed was a torrent of apocalyptic imaginings—a social contagion—that cascaded through many national populations. This tidal

Table 2.9 IHME projected mean hospital COVID-19 beds needed vs actual COVID-19 serious and critical care hospitalisations, United States

IHME COVID-19 estimates, mean COVID-19 Beds Needed			Actual Serious and Critical Care Hospitalisations
March 25 release	April 1 release	April 8 release	
March 15 Projected 3503	March 15 Projected 3922	March 15 Projected 1338	March 15 Actual 10
March 30 Projected 96,733	March 30 Projected 93,743	March 30 Projected 36,646	March 30 Actual 1411
April 11 Projected 226,620	April 11 Projected 246,346	April 11 Projected 94,248	April 11 Actual 11,320
April 26 Projected 166,643	April 26 Projected 204,571	April 28 Projected 55,754	April 26 Actual 15,143

Sources: IHME, Institute for Health Metrics and Evaluation, COVID-19 estimate downloads, http://www.healthdata.org/covid/data-downloads; Worldometer Coronavirus daily reports by country, USA, Internet Archive https://www.worldometers.info/coronavirus/

wave of "imagining the worst" was reinforced by obsessive daily case and death counts. But was the COVID episode actually an apocalypse? Or was it a serious mid-range public health matter that then was blown out of all proportion? In Europe as death tolls associated with COVID-19 grew through March and April and reached a peak in April 2020, measures of excess deaths [rate of deaths greater than what would normally be expected] indicated that the matter was serious but variable in its seriousness and far from apocalyptic—and confined to a relatively short time period as would be expected from the bell-curve pattern of viral pandemics (Tables 1.2 and 1.3). Yet forebodings of immanent disaster circulated widely even while the worst death rates per capita were confined to specific nations and even in those cases to regional hotspots (Tables 1.10 and 1.11).

2.2 The Ferguson Report

The report for the British government produced in March 2020 by Imperial College, London, researchers led by Professor Neil Ferguson (hereafter the Ferguson report or the Imperial College report) was the

2 PUBLIC POLICY

Table 2.10 Comparison of the projected loss of life-span years from COVID-19 deaths [Imperial College model] with the loss of life-span years from unemployment in a major recession, United Kingdom

R_0	On Trigger	Do Nothing Total Deaths	Projected total life span years lost from CV deaths	Total life span years lost from recession with 10% unemployment peak	CV life span years lost + or − recession life span years lost	CI_HQ_SD Total Deaths	Projected total life span years lost from CV deaths	Total life span years lost from recession with 10% unemployment peak	CV life span years lost + or − recession life span years lost
2	60	410,000	2,788,000	3,275,000	−487,000	47,000	319,600	3,275,000	−2,955,400
2.2	100	460,000	3,128,000	3,275,000	−147,000	61,000	414,800	3,275,000	−2,860,200
2.4	300	510,000	3,468,000	3,275,000	193,000	94,000	639,200	3,275,000	−2,635,800
2.6	400	550,000	3,740,000	3,275,000	465,000	120,000	816,000	3,275,000	−2,459,000
R_0	On Trigger	PC_CI_SD Total Deaths				PC_CI_HQ_SD Total Deaths			
2	60	6400	43,520	3,275,000	−3,231,480	5600	38,080	3,275,000	−3,236,920
2.2	100	13,000	88,400	3,275,000	−3,186,600	10,000	68,000	3,275,000	−3,207,000
2.4	300	43,000	292,400	3,275,000	−2,982,600	34,000	231,200	3,275,000	−3,043,800
2.6	400	48,000	326,400	3,275,000	−2,948,600	48,000	326,400	3,275,000	−2,948,600

Notes: UK workforce: 32.75 million (ONS, July 2019)

UK projected Second Quarter 2020 unemployment rate: "Unemployment rises by more than 2 million to 10 per cent in the second quarter, but then declines more slowly than GDP recovers." UK Office of Budget Responsibility, 14 April 2020

Projected UK GDP growth contraction in 2020: −6.5 percent (IMF, World Economic Outlook, April 2020, Table 1.1)

Note: The estimate of the loss of life span years through the experience of mass unemployment (1 year per displaced employee) is derived from (a) Sullivan, D. & Till Wachter, T.V. (2009) Job Displacement and Mortality: An Analysis Using Administrative Data, The Quarterly Journal of Economics, Table V, 1289. The study was based on "administrative data on the quarterly employment and earnings of Pennsylvanian workers in the 1970s and 1980s matched to

(*continued*)

Table 2.10 (continued)

Social Security Administration death records covering 1980–2006". Sullian and Wachter concluded that the bust-era cohort of unemployed workers with three or five years in a job and aged 30–55 at the time of displacement lost an average of 1.5 life span years compared with employees who were not displaced; (b) Schwandt, H. & Wachter, T.V. (2019, October) Socioeconomic Decline and Death: Midlife Impacts of Graduating in a Recession [later, NBER Working Paper No. 26638, January 2020], an analysis of new entrants into the US 1982 labor market "facing a 3.9 percentage point increase in the entry unemployment rate", concludes that new labor market entrants in a mass layoff era lose between 5.9 and 8.9 months of life expectancy per person

Note 2: The table assumes the average age of those who die is 79 years old (Italian National Institute of Health, 17 March 2020) and that they have on average three chronic health conditions (UK Office of National Statistics, Deaths involving COVID-19, England and Wales: deaths occurring in March 2020). It is further assumed that the life expectancy of a person aged 79 years with three pre-existing chronic conditions is 6.8 years, an estimate based on the American study by DuGoff, E.H. et al. (2014) Multiple Chronic Conditions and Life Expectancy A Life Table Analysis, Medical Care, 52(8)

Imperial College Model, Impact of non-pharmaceutical interventions (NPIs) to reduce COVID-19 mortality and healthcare demand, 16 March 2020, abbreviations:

R_0 Basic Reproduction Number, or the number of persons a single person will infect with the virus

Triggers: public policy interventions trigged by numbers of critical care [ICU] cases

CI Case isolation in the home: Symptomatic cases stay at home for 7 days, reducing non-household contacts by 75% for this period. Household contacts remain unchanged. Assume 70% of household comply with the policy

HQ Voluntary home quarantine: Following identification of a symptomatic case in the household, all household members remain at home for 14 days. Household contact rates double during this quarantine period, contacts in the community reduce by 75%. Assume 50% of household comply with the policy

SDO Social distancing of those over 70 years of age: Reduce contacts by 50% in workplaces, increase household contacts by 25% and reduce other contacts by 75%. Assume 75% compliance with policy

SD Social distancing of entire population: All households reduce contact outside household, school or workplace by 75%. School contact rates unchanged, workplace contact rates reduced by 25%. Household contact rates assumed to increase by 25%. *SD* assumed effectively a national lockdown of the population.

PC Closure of schools and universities: Closure of all schools, 25% of universities remain open. Household contact rates for student families increase by 50% during closure. Contacts in the community increase by 25% during closure

Source: Ferguson, N.M. et al. (2020, March 16) Impact of non-pharmaceutical interventions (NPIs) to reduce COVID-19 mortality and healthcare demand

single most influential document produced during the COVID-19 episode (Ferguson et al. 2020, March 16). Its influence was enormous. It galvanized governments (not just in the United Kingdom but more generally) to impose increasingly severe shutdown policies. The paper gave different estimates of total deaths over a five month or longer period depending on different reproduction numbers and different "suppression strategies" (Table 2.10). Among an enormous range of predictions of total deaths in the UK—ranging from 500,000 to 5600—the report had to make some more or less correct predictions almost by definition. In a way the model couldn't be wrong—or usefully right. The modelling of the number of American deaths by the Institute for Health Metrics and Evaluation at the University of Washington proved much more reliable not least because its numbers concentrated on the mean projected number of fatalities—a notable step in the direction of statistical humility (Table 2.11).

Modelling of future behaviour and effects is based on assumptions and parameters. Where such assumptions and parameters (at least 400 of them in the case of Ferguson report) work well is when the phenomenon being modelled is a known quantity whose behaviour and effects has been previously empirically observed and recorded. Assumptions then can be made on the basis of what has happened in reality. The problem with a novel entity, such as COVID-19, is that the assumptions of a model are unlikely

Table 2.11 IHME projected mean cumulative COVID-19 deaths vs actual COVID-19 deaths, United States

IHME COVID-19 estimates, deaths, mean projected			Actual Deaths
March 25 release	April 1 release	April 8 release	
March 15 Projected 79	March 15 Projected 79	March 15 Projected 79	March 15 Actual 68
March 30 Projected 3182	March 30 Projected 2997	March 30 Projected 2997	March 30 Actual 931
April 11 Projected 22,297	April 11 Projected 22,253	April 11 Projected 20,899	April 11 Actual 20,562
April 26 Projected 53,865	April 26 Projected 59,119	April 26 Projected 47,997	April 26 Actual 55,415

Sources: IHME, Institute for Health Metrics and Evaluation, COVID-19 estimate downloads, http://www.healthdata.org/covid/data-downloads; Worldometer Coronavirus daily reports by country, USA, Internet Archive https://www.worldometers.info/coronavirus/

to capture how the virus actually behaves in reality. How could a model created in March 2020 anticipate the possibility of research in May 2020 that suggested that a body's established ability to fight the "common cold" coronaviruses might adapt itself to fight the COVID-19 virus which also is a species of coronavirus (Grifoni et al. 2020, May 7)? Assume the latter is true for a moment. It has all kinds of implications for the potential deadliness of the virus and the susceptibility of the population to the virus. Without a weighty empirical anchor, a model may be little more than fiction.

As far as the social dimension of the behaviour of COVID-19 is concerned, the largest blind-spot in the Ferguson report to government was its failure to adequately identify the discriminating nature of the virus and highlight the implications of this. The lacuna itself subdivides into three subsidiary lacunae:

Firstly, the Ferguson report noted the way the virus targeted different age groups and noted in passing the significance of pre-existing health conditions. The virus was most lethal for the over seventies and eighties, and those with chronic underlying health conditions, and especially those over seventies and eighties with underlying serious health conditions. Yet the highly targeted nature of the virus' behaviour was not reflected in the report's "whole of population" policy prescriptions that, in effect, treated the entire population as at high risk of either transmitting the virus or being exposed to the virus or dying from the virus.

Secondly, the Ferguson report did not discuss the significance of or draw policy conclusions from one of the key pattern behaviours of the virus: the relatively narrow band of social contact that the virus typically was transmitted through. This was a spectrum of persons predominately composed of family (spouses not children), relatives, friends and acquaintances in physically close contact and usually for a prolonged period.

Thirdly, the Ferguson report did not identify that the spread of the virus varied remarkably between region, city and nation—and even within cities. The viral spread was not a uniform phenomenon that required or demanded or was best served by uniform solutions. The cognitive bias of public health officials is toward uniform regulation and prohibition. This bias is echoed in the Ferguson report. Universal law allows a lot of flexibility. Uniform regulations do not. The recommended Ferguson policies focused on the nation as a single entity. But the virus behaved regionally not nationally. Even within regions clusters occurred. The virus had a

highly differentiated impact globally which was repeated nationally, regionally and sub-regionally in a fractal-like manner.
Three examples illustrate the point:

(a) Consider the results for national serological testing (testing for herd immunity antibodies to the virus) in mid-May 2020 (these are a snap-shot of the past, as anti-bodies take almost three weeks to form in the human body from symptom onset) (Long et al. 2020). Spain's infection spread was estimated by serological testing to be 5% (López 2020). But the regional differences hidden beneath this headline figure were telling. Madrid's rate of infection was 15%. Barcelona's was 8%. At the national level, France's spread was calculated at 4.4%.[8] But in the Paris region it was 9.9% and in Grand Est 9.1%. In Sweden, 7.3% of the population in Stockholm had been exposed to the virus compared to 4.2% in provincial Skåne (Anon 2020b, May 20).

(b) Similar heterogeneity is evident in the UK, as we can see from the spectrum of cumulative cases (per 100,000 population) in different cities as of 13 May 2020. The differences are striking: Portsmouth (144), Bristol (147), Richmond on Thames* (203), Leeds (212), Hackney* (223), Birmingham (281), Liverpool (307), Luton (311), Newcastle upon Tyne (333), Ealing* (335), Southend on Sea (346), Sheffield (418), South Tyneside (457) and Sunderland (481).[9] Urban density played no role in this hierarchy of case incidence as is evident when we look at the population density (persons per square kilometre) of the same sequence of cities: Portsmouth (5326), Bristol (4224), Richmond on Thames (3430), Leeds (1430), Hackney (14,681), Birmingham (4262), Liverpool (4242), Luton (4939), Newcastle upon Tyne (2646), Ealing (6157), Southend on Sea (4370), Sheffield (1583), South Tyneside (2334) and Sunderland (2018).[10]

(c) Perhaps the most striking examples of the heterogeneous impact of the virus was the policy of lockdown itself. Numerous countries adopted official lockdown policies. Yet the results of policies that were the same or similar were markedly divergent. If we are to assume that lockdown policies had an effect—that is they had some kind of causal power—then that should be evident in the spread and fatality of the virus. All countries applied some government controls (such as border controls or banning entertainment establishments). But not all countries had government-mandated stay-at-home policies. Yet through the months of April and May 2020, lockdown (stay-at-home) countries covered the entire spectrum from low morbidity per capita countries like Australia to high deaths per capita countries like the United Kingdom, Italy and Spain. The same applied to no lockdown countries. Iceland, Taiwan, Hong Kong, South Korea, Japan, Latvia and Estonia had low or relatively low rates of morbidity per capita while Sweden's rate was relatively high.[11]

The fact that several countries avoided lockdown *and* achieved a low per capita rate of death strongly implies that government stay-at-home prohibitions shutting down large parts of a nation's economy and society were not actually necessary to reduce the effective reproduction rate of the disease. The point is not that government controls had no positive benefits. Every country deployed such controls. But that government action—or rather its efficacy—had limits. Yet the Imperial College model assumed that there were only two effective causal agents: government policy and the viral agent itself. Meaningful action was equated with government action. The tacit principle of the Imperial College researchers was that the only effective counter to the virus was the mandated shutting down of much of a country's economic and social activity. This required much of the population to stay-at-home, and (where practical) work-from-home along with the closing of much of a country's face-to-face businesses and outlets excepting those deemed "essential".

As it turned out, the potency of the viral agent varied more according to social conditions than government proscription. Government action could modulate social patterns to a degree. But it could not control, create or erase such patterns. The Imperial College report supposed a causal power of government to modify both viral and social agency—and their interrelationship—to a degree that it did not and could not possess. The potency of the virus varied according to the age of persons exposed to it and their underlying health condition. Crucially though, in addition to that, the effects of the virus varied according to patterns of social connection—cultural and social patterns of everyday proximity and haptics and preferred psychological space. These patterns encapsulated habitual, deeply-encoded, micro-logically structured and historically-formed modes of social closeness and distance.

A study drawn on by the Ferguson paper estimated a virus infection fatality rate of 0.66% based on Chinese data concerning 3665 cases (Verity et al. 2020, March 13, p. 8). The Ferguson paper upped the IFR estimate to 0.9% by assuming a set of age-stratified estimates of IFR, notably that 9.3% of infected persons aged 80 and over would die from the infection along with 5.1% of those aged 70–79 compared to 0.002% of 0–9 year olds (Ferguson et al. 2020, p. 5). The Ferguson paper thus assumed that age was a major variable factor in the impact of the virus, as it proved to be. But it is notable that in the Imperial College paper there is no explicit reference to significant countervailing social factors reducing infection exposure—at least none stated to be effective—except for broad-spectrum government intervention (shutdown).

2.3 Mitigation

In the Imperial College model two strategies only were laid out (Ferguson et al. 2020, p. 3). One was to *mitigate* the virus via the "home isolation of suspect cases, home quarantine of those living in the same household as suspect cases, and social distancing of the elderly and others at most risk of severe disease". The second was to *suppress* the virus. The first strategy could only slow the spread of the virus, the model argued. Unlike the second strategy, it could not reduce the virus reproduction number below 1. Suppression was the result exclusively of government-mandated actions. The model of China was explicitly cited by the Ferguson paper. "Through the hospitalisation of all cases (not just those requiring hospital care), China in effect initiated a form of case isolation, reducing onward transmission from cases in the household and in other settings. At the same time, by implementing population-wide social distancing, the opportunity for onward transmission in all locations was rapidly reduced. Several studies have estimated that these interventions reduced R to below 1" (Ferguson et al. 2020, p. 14). One study published on February 18 2020—by researchers in the Centre for Mathematical Modelling of Infectious Diseases in the London School of Hygiene and Tropical Medicine—was cited by the Imperial College researchers. The Ferguson report summarised it as concluding that the median daily reproduction number declined from 2.35 one week before the Chinese government introduced travel restrictions in Wuhan on January 23 to 1.05 on January 31.[12] From that one statistic in one report attributed to one act of Chinese government control in Hubei province, the Imperial College researchers concluded that government control was the key to management of the virus. The causality for the drop that occurred in the effective reproduction number was implied though it was not demonstrated. It is notable however that it was January 26 when the death rate from the virus peaked in Hubei Province, indicating that infections in the region had peaked three weeks *before* the Chinese government action, as the virus developed conventionally along a bell-curve path.[13]

In the UK context, "population-wide social distancing" meant the closing of schools, churches, bars and social events. The Imperial College researchers' virus suppression strategy assumed that all households would reduce contact outside household, school or workplace by 75%, workplace contact rates would be reduced by 25% and household contact rates were assumed to increase by 25% (Ferguson et al., Table 2). This advice to government, made on March 16 2020, was directly at odds with the scope and tenor of the recommendations for antiviral measures that were made by the British government's SAGE (Scientific Advisory Group for Emergencies) Committee from its first COVID meeting on January 22 2020 right up until the pivotal March 16 date.[14] Between March 13 and March 16 it is evident from the SAGE Committee's minutes that, during those few days, the exogenous force of nervous public opinion and the British government's own evidently spooked response to both the virus and public pressure had the effect of over-determining what had been previously the Committee's generally sober, realistic and evidence-based approach (SAGE 2020).

Prior to the March 16, the SAGE Committee had recommended the following as measures to mitigate the virus: port-of-entry screening only if a simple and rapid test was available (January 22), self-isolation of infected persons (January 28), infection control in healthcare settings (January 28), and the rapid detection of cases (January 28). SAGE allowed itself various "assumptions"—namely, that the reproduction number of the virus was between 2 and 3 (January 22, January 28, February 11) and the virus was similar to an influenza (January 28, February 4, February 11). The Committee's forecasts of the peak of the Wuhan/Hubei infections were badly wrong (February 4, February 11) as was its March 10 projection of the UK peak. Earlier, more accurately, it estimated that the peak of UK infections would occur 2–3 months after widespread transmission began (February 11). Also to its credit, the Committee repeatedly asked for more empirical data and serological testing to establish the virus' actual spread in the community as opposed to its spread modelled on "assumptions". To understand the epidemic, it was important to have case numbers reported by their onset date, data on numbers of people being tested, the age distribution of cases and co-morbidity information (February 3). The Committee noted it was significant that, as of February 4, there had been no reports of illness among children, under-20s appeared to be least susceptible and most deaths were among the over-60s (see also February 11). Serological evidence was the best means of predicting an epidemiological peak (February 20) and determining the ratio of asymptomatic to symptomatic cases (March 16).

The SAGE Committee was appropriately sceptical about many of the measures suggested to control the virus. A 95% effective ban on travel to the UK would not supress the virus, only delay its impact by a month (February 3). Shutting down public transport (February 4, February 11, March 18) or restricting public gatherings (February 4, February 11, March 3, March 5) or travel restrictions within the UK (February 11) would be ineffective in delaying the spread of the virus. School closures would only have a modest impact on delaying the peak of the virus (February 20, March 5). At best the effect of these closures was "uncertain" (March 18). Implying the lack of any prior empirical evidence, the Committee noted that modelling could not analyse with "great precision" the impact of closing schools, restaurants, bars, entertainment, indoor public places or indoor workplaces (March 18).

On February 25 the SAGE Committee speculated that a four-step mitigation policy of school closures, home isolation, home quarantine and the social distancing of the elderly could reduce the reproduction number of the virus below 1. This policy outline was fashioned after the experience of Wuhan, Hong Kong and Singapore. The Committee also hinted at homeworking for businesses. On March 3 the Committee noted that "social distancing for over-65s is likely to have a significant effect on overall deaths and peak demand for critical care beds" even if this would "not significantly reduce overall transmission". By March 5 (and subsequently on March 10 and March 13) these ideas were boiled down to an anti-virus plan with three components: home isolation of symptomatic persons, isolation of infected households and the cocooning (social distancing) of over-65s and those with underlying medical conditions. The latter advice was refined on March 10. "SAGE agreed that social distancing measures for the elderly should apply to those aged 70+." The "cocooning" of persons was relevant to two distinct groups: "a) those aged 70+ who are generally well and b) vulnerable groups of all ages (including those aged 70+)". There was, the Committee added, limited evidence that children were at risk from the virus. Children, the Committee observed, will "mostly experience mild illness, though they probably transmit the virus".

On March 13 and 18 the SAGE Committee stated it was keen to make its modelling and other inputs underpinning its advice available to the public and fellow scientists. The political wind though was blowing in the opposite direction. The British government led by Prime Minister Boris Johnson proved reluctant to release the SAGE minutes. It did so only after a court case forced its hand. In reality the government was tracking away from SAGE's tailored and circumspect recommendations. On March 16, the Ferguson report was released. It concluded that the SAGE mitigation measures "might reduce peak healthcare demand by 2/3 and deaths by half". However "the resulting mitigated epidemic would still likely result in hundreds of thousands of deaths and health systems (most notably intensive care units) being overwhelmed many times over" (Ferguson et al. 2020, p. 1). The Ferguson estimate of deaths resulting from the mitigation strategy is empirically testable. Uppsala University researchers applied the Ferguson model to Sweden (Gardner et al. 2020). Sweden's public health model relied on a largely self-managing mitigation model. In April 2020 the Uppsala researchers predicted that Sweden's public health model would result in a median projected mortality of 96,000 (somewhere between 52,000 and 183,000 deaths) by July 1, 2020. With SAGE-like mitigation policies that outcome, they estimated, would be reduced to 48,000 deaths (26,000–91,500). As of June 14, Sweden had a total of 4874 COVID-related deaths.

If the government of Boris Johnson had ever committed itself to a mitigation strategy, the Ferguson report effectively put an end to that. On March 16, the SAGE Committee reiterated its social distancing measures. It repeated that school closures were not a particularly effective measure. It conceded that closing schools might be a measure needed to keep demand for critical care hospital beds at a viable level. But its scepticism about school closures was still clearly evident—as it was again on March 18 when it reiterated that the evidence about the effect of school closures was "uncertain". The Committee though agreed that "its advice on interventions should be based on what the NHS needs" (March 16)—a telltale sign of what was then emerging in the United Kingdom and elsewhere, namely a view that the priority in fighting the virus was to protect the nation's hospital system. In any event the modelling of apocalyptic population and institutional scenarios decisively overshadowed more proportionate measures that were tailored to the known empirical behaviour of the virus whose impact overwhelmingly was on the over-70s and those with underlying chronic conditions. Instead only the shut-down of Britain's society and economy with stay-at-home orders directed at schools, businesses and organizations could stop the apocalypse of hundreds of thousands of deaths, a scenario that was modelled on the behaviour of influenza—a virus whose profile was significantly unlike that of the COVID-19 virus.

In the absence of any government control measures or spontaneous social behavioural changes—that is, if society and government did nothing at all—the Ferguson report estimated that the R number of the virus would remain at around 2.4 and 81% of the population would be infected before the virus petered out due to community immunity. *Only* government control would bring the R number down below 1. However, Gomes et al. (2020, May 2) suggested that social variation or population heterogeneity places considerably more downward pressure on viral behaviour than the Ferguson model allowed for. As the Gomes paper observed, *variation in individual susceptibility* to the virus (e.g. the age of a person or their underlying chronic health status) affects the rate at which new cases occur as does crucially *variation in exposure* to the virus (for example degrees of closeness of physical contact). Populations, in other words, are heterogeneous in nature—and not just in terms of age. The coefficient of variation is a statistical measure of relative variability. It is the measure of the ratio of the standard deviation of data points to the mean. Gomes (et al.) searched existing literature for estimates of individual variation in the propensity to acquire or transmit COVID-19. Most coefficient of variation estimates, they concluded, were between 2 and 4. This was a range, they observed, where naturally acquired immunity to COVID-19 might place a population over the "herd immunity" threshold once as few as 10–20% of its individuals were immune.[15] It should be remembered in this context that the 1918 Spanish flu—more virulent than COVID-19—infected 30% of the world's population and then dissipated.[16] The cruise ship, the *Diamond Princess*, was a living laboratory for the interaction of COVID-19 with a human population. 3700 passengers and crew in an enclosed and close-contact environment were exposed for a month in February 2020 to the risk of acquiring COVID-19. Eventually 19.2% of this population were infected. The Imperial College estimate was that, without stern government intervention, 80% of the UK population would eventually be infected mostly over a two month period before abating.[17] This implied a community immunity threshold of 50–60%, which was also the most common reported expectation of virologists, epidemiologists and other specialists at the start of the epidemic.

The Ferguson paper made explicit age as a factor responsible for a significant variation in individual susceptibility to the virus and hinted at underlying health conditions as a further factor. But what about variation in exposure to the virus? The propensity of a person to be exposed is at least in part social and cultural in nature.[18] The closeness and distance in interaction between persons—and whether droplets can pass effectively between an infected person and a susceptible person—is a cultural and social phenomenon, one that is pervasive in human relationships. But throughout the Imperial College paper the word "social", which recurs, is almost exclusively used in conjunction with government action—whether the action is to close schools, churches, bars and similar venues or else to mandate by regulation the social distancing of "the whole population". Any projected or preferred social action is closely entangled with government-directed "population-wide" measures. There was not only an implicit and explicit link made between "the social" and "the governmental"—which in itself is not unreasonable—but in addition to this it was assumed, almost unconsciously, that government was not just *an* active agent in shaping social behaviour but *the only* active agent.

Socially distancing of "the whole population" in contrast to virus mitigation strategies assumed that the everyday interaction of strangers or semi-strangers constituted high-risk behaviour. But the converse was true. The more intimate the social connection the higher the risk simply because the principal transmission of the virus was via families, relatives, friends and acquaintances. Not strangers in public transport, at work or in hospital settings but interactions with intimates—be it at home, travelling on public transport together or elsewhere. Not the solo walker in the national park or the lonely jogger on the sidewalk but dyads and triads and larger groups of friends, families, relatives and friendly acquaintances.

The Imperial College report cited a study of close contacts in the spread of infectious diseases that noted that the large differences (the heterogeneity) in physicality depending on the type of social interaction. It observed that "contacts lasting at least one hour or occurring on a daily basis mostly involved physical contact, while short duration and infrequent contacts tended to be nonphysical. Contacts at home, school, or leisure were more likely to be physical than contacts at the workplace or while travelling" (Mossong et al. 2020).[19] The World Health Organization (WHO) in February reported that household transmission was the primary conduit for the virus.[20] The Imperial College report noted this but also downplayed its significance on the grounds that this had occurred in a context where social contact had been markedly reduced by government intervention (Ferguson et al. 2020, p. 15). This was stated even though cluster studies in China included the tracing and cataloguing of infection cases that occurred *before* Chinese government intervention in late January. Many if not most of the cases in the studies that were reported to WHO visitors in the third week of February would have been infected *before* the Chinese government lockdown. And the primacy of household transmission was confirmed in country studies outside China where shutdown had not occurred or had not yet occurred (Cheng et al. 2020, May 1; Ghinai et al. 2020, March 13).

2.4 UNINTENDED CONSEQUENCES

Is social distancing of "a whole population" a proportionate response to a virus that reproduces itself primary through household and related close physical contact such as in nursing homes? Such a strategy will reduce social contact in the public sphere dramatically—though it also increases household contact. But is public interaction—the interaction of strangers—really an appropriate target to manage a virus whose mode of transmission is primarily intimate or personal but not public? Also is public interaction an appropriate target when, as the Imperial College researchers noted in passing, it means high economic and social costs? Is reducing the interaction of strangers and near-strangers in a broad-spectrum—essentially unselective and undiscriminating—manner prudent if it means shutting down much of a society's economic and business activity and shutting persons in their homes with predictable increases in depression and anxiety—and long-term reductions in life-span years for persons most severely affected by any resulting economic downturn (Table 2.10)?

The shutdown of society and economy became commonplace throughout the world in April 2020. The intensity of the shutdowns varied between nations (Tables 2.3 and 2.4). The immediate economic impact across the board was variable but typically severe (Tables 2.12 and 2.13). As for the longer-term impact of COVID policies on economies, it is not an easy thing to predict the outcome of what were in effect government-engineered recessions because there is no precedent for them. In April 2020 the International Monetary Fund (IMF) forecast a -6.6% real GDP decline among the economically advanced European nations and a 9.2%

Table 2.12 Purchasing Managers Index (PMI), manufacturing by country, expansion and contraction

Country	April 2020	March 2020	February 2020	November 2019	February 2019
Spain	30.8	45.7	50.4	47.5	49.9
Italy	31.1	40.3	48.7	47.6	47.7
France	15.0	43.2	49.7	51.7	51.5
Netherlands	41.3	50.5	52.9	49.6	52.7
Switzerland	40.7	43.7	49.5	48.5	54.3
United Kingdom	32.9	47.8	51.7	48.9	52.1
Sweden	36.7	43.2	53.2	46.4	52
Denmark	38.6	46.8	49.1	53.6	61.5
United States	36.9	48.5	50.7	52.6	53
Germany	34.4	45.5	48	44.1	47.6
Canada	33.0	46.1	51.8	51.4	52.6
South Korea	41.6	44.2	44.4	49.4	47.2
China	49.4	50.1	40.3	51.8	49.9
Australia	45.6	49.7	50.1	49.9	53.1
Singapore	44.7	45.4	48.7	49.8	50.4
Japan	43.7	44.8	47.8	48.9	48.9
Hong Kong	36.9	34.9	33.1	38.5	48.4
Taiwan	42.2	50.4	49.9	49.8	46.3

Source: The Global Economy, Purchasing Managers Index (PMI), manufacturing by country, April 30 2020

Note: >50 = expansion; <50 = contraction; Based on a survey of business as to whether their supplier deliveries, inventory levels, production, employment and new orders are expanding, contracting or staying the same. Each factor is equally weighted

unemployment rate in 2020 (IMF 2020). In the major economies of Asia, the projected figures were -4.5% GDP growth and 4.1% unemployment. Advanced economies predicted to have 10% or more unemployment in 2020 included Germany, France, Italy, Spain, Ireland, Portugal, Greece, Sweden, Norway, and the United States. As of April 29, many major economies had borrowed heavily to provide economic stimulus packages to sustain economies that had been furloughed during lockdowns until they could restart once shutdown measures were eased or removed. In the case of Germany the government stimulus package was the equivalent of 18.2% of GDP; Japan 14.3%; the United States 13.6%; Australia 12.9%; France 9.5%; Italy 8.5%; South Korea 8.1%; Canada 6.3% and China 3.7% (Segal and Gerstel 2020).[21]

Table 2.13 Purchasing Managers Index (PMI), services by country, expansion and contraction

Country	April 2020	March 2020	February 2020	November 2019	February 2019
Spain	7.1	23.0	52.1	53.2	54.5
Italy	10.8	17.4	52.1	50.4	50.4
France	10.4	27.4	52.6	52.5	50.2
Switzerland	21.4	44.7	51.9	52.6	56.2
United Kingdom	12.3	35.7	53.2	49.3	51.3
Sweden	39.0	46.9	56.7	48.2	55.3
United States	27.0	39.8	49.4	51.6	56.0
Germany	16.2	31.7	52.5	51.7	55.3
China	44.4	40.3	26.5	53.5	51.1
Australia	19.5	38.5	49.0	49.7	48.7
Japan	21.5	33.8	46.8	50.3	52.3

Source: The Global Economy, Purchasing Managers Index (PMI), services by country, April 302,020

Note: >50 = expansion; <50 = contraction; Based on a survey of business as to whether their supplier deliveries, inventory levels, production, employment and new orders are expanding, contracting or staying the same. Each factor is equally weighted

Social life is multi-dimensional. It requires the balancing of multiple private and public goods. A sense of proportionate behaviour is necessary to accompany this. One cannot with justification elevate one good without taking into consideration other competing goods. Proportionality is crucial. In a given time period we might treat an issue like the spread of a pathogen as "serious". So a certain proportion of time and resources is devoted to it. 60:40 might be an appropriate weighting. Let us call this an Aristotelian approach to public policy. It assumes that there is a "middle way" in public policy—a balancing of competing considerations. Good judgment—or prudence—is the intellectual virtue that reflects this. Good judgment is different from the notion of the need to act out of "an abundance of caution" that was common in government statements during late March and April 2020. This supposes that governments can eliminate risk from societies caught-up in a state of uncertainty. This is impossible. Attempting to entirely eliminate one risk creates other, even greater, risks as a result. What is the right relation to risk? It's not fear. Nor is it foolhardiness. Rather it's prudence. In making prudential judgments we take risk into account and modify behaviour accordingly. But we don't cave into fears and anxieties.

Rushing urgently in one direction to avoid a risk may lead unintentionally to other equally bad or worse outcomes from other unseen risks. Take the case of deaths—specifically the number of excess deaths per week by country in March, April and May 2020 (Table 1.2). Tallies of excess deaths allow us to calculate the number of deaths attributable to COVID-19 separate from COVID-related deaths due principally to co-morbidities. The question though is: attributable to COVID-19 in what way? A percentage of persons exposed to the virus will die directly as a result of that exposure. But among excess deaths there are also deaths of persons with no infection that were caused by anti-COVID public policy measures. It has long been observed that public policy routinely leads to (negative) unintended consequences. Take the case of England and Wales. Between Week 1 and Week 11 of 2020 these regions had below average deaths (-4894) compared with their five year average.[22] Between Week 12 and Week 19, deaths substantially exceeded the weekly five year average by 49,647 deaths. Of those though 37,290 were COVID related, leaving an additional 12,357 deaths to be accounted for.

Researchers examining population-based health records in England and Northern Ireland found that, during the public health emergency period, there was a 44–66% drop in admissions for chemotherapy and a 70–89% reduction in urgent referrals for early cancer diagnosis compared to pre-emergency levels (Lai et al. 2020). They calculated that this represented, in its effects on mortality, 6270 excess deaths at 1 year in England and 33,890 excess deaths in the US. The British Heart Foundation reported that in March 2020 the number of people in England attending emergency departments with the symptoms of a possible heart attack dropped from an average of around 300 per day at the start of the month to around 150 per day at the end of the month (Bakker 2020, April 9). Coronary heart disease is the top cause of death in the United Kingdom, accounting for around 16% (96,000) of the 600,000 persons who die in the UK annually.

In the United States, by April 7, 261 hospitals (4%) had furloughed employees because of declining admissions and the related suspension of elective procedures due to the COVID episode (Paavola 2020). Consumer spending on healthcare in the US fell by 18% in the first quarter of 2020 (Coombs 2020, April 29).[23] A research study found an increase in observed, compared with expected, mortality in Scotland (+73%), England

and Wales (+49%), the Netherlands (+65%) and New York state (+34%).[24] But of these deaths, only 65% in Scotland, 68% in England and Wales, 49% in the Netherlands and 73% in New York State were attributable to COVID-19 infections. How to explain the number of excess deaths that were not attributable to COVID-19 infections? COVID public policy measures and associated rhetoric disrupted normal clinical patterns. Populations avoided emergency, medical and hospital waiting rooms because of stay-at-home pressures and fears of infection. The effect was a pronounced fall in the diagnosis and treatment of life-threatening non-COVID conditions.[25]

The unintended consequences of public policy span not only the short term but also the long term. Governments paid close attention to the projected loss of life-span due to COVID-19 but did not give proportionate attention to the significantly larger number of life-span years lost when societies are plunged (or in this case plunge themselves) into periods of mass unemployment (Table 2.10). Prudent social distancing to reduce the R_E number of the virus would have led to global recession in any event by slowing and curbing social interaction but not nearly to the same degree as government stay-at-home orders. The greater the degree of shut-down, the larger the unintended negative effects on physical and mental health.

Economies are robust. They bounce back after recessions. But, as probable in the case of COVID-19, a major recession in economic activity means a period of time with as much as 10% unemployment. This is not just an economic phenomenon. It is also a health phenomenon. What follows eventually from periods of high unemployment are deaths of despair—or, in a more technical sense, shorter life-spans for those who were out of work for significant periods of time.[26] The psychological and mental dynamics that lead to this are well-known and set out in Table 2.14. A prudent balanced approach to public policy would consider deaths in the long-term as well as the short-term. Not least, as in the case of COVID-19, when the long-term loss of life-span years (assuming a mass 10% unemployment peak) far outweighs any but the most extreme COVID-19 mortality scenarios (Table 2.10).

The remarkable thing about the public policy decisions to shutter economies in late March and April 2020 is how little cost-benefit analysis was applied to the process. There was almost a complete absence of balance in public policy making during this period. Public policy routinely deals with competing goods. Any major government action involves trade-offs. The opportunity to do X always comes with Y cost. Resources devoted to A

Table 2.14 Near-term visible expressions of long-term pathways to deaths of despair

Despair: "sentiment affecting entire segments of a population in response to the bleak conditions that follow economic stagnation"

Forms of despair

Cognitive despair

Thoughts indicating defeat, hopelessness, guilt, worthlessness, learned helplessness, pessimism, and limited positive expectations for the future

Cognitive biases including repeated mistakes in perceiving, interpreting, and remembering others' actions as antagonistic (e.g., hostile attribution bias)

Hyperbolic discounting: giving undue weight to current outcomes and discounting the value of longterm outcomes; assuming the long-term future may never come to pass

Depressed thoughts of resignation, defeat; anxious thoughts

Emotional despair

Feelings of excessive sadness, irritability, hostility or loneliness

Anhedonia and apathy: the inability to experience pleasure and reward and the resulting lack of motivation and action

Behavioral despair

Risky, reckless or unhealthy acts that are self-destructive and reflect limited hope for the future

Examples: high-risk sexual behaviors, gambling, self-harm, reckless driving, excessive spending, criminal activity, smoking, substance use, low physical activity

Inaction, learned helplessness, sickness behaviors

Biological despair

The body's stress reactive systems no longer function homeostatically and show signs of dysregulation or depletion

Biological despair manifests itself in the hypothalamic–pituitary–adrenal axis, the autonomous nervous system, and the immune system

Biological despair can be inferred from changes in body functions (e.g., sleep, appetite, concentration or restlessness, and somatic symptoms or pain)

Social despair

Arises in networks and communities when their members are exposed to the same distressing event

Social contagion: the diffusion of (or increasing similarity in) emotions, cognition, behavior, or biology in social contexts

Pathways to deaths of despair

Increase in *despair in different domains* leads to *diseases of despair* (suicidal ideation and attempts, illicit drug use, alcohol abuse and addiction) leads to increased risks of deaths of despair, and autoimmune and infectious diseases

Source: Shanahan, L. et al. (2019) Does Despair Really Kill? A Roadmap for an Evidence-Based Answer, American Journal of Public Health AJPH Perspectives, January 26

cannot be allocated to Z. Yet in late March and April there was no concentrated public discussion of the costs and benefits of an Imperial College-style shutdown approach. There was no discussion of whether the projected decrease (a speculative outcome at best) in the virus' reproduction number could justify a 6% drop in annual economic growth in 2020 (even offset by a 4% rebound in growth in 2021). Nor was there clear and compelling evidence presented that extreme artificial social distancing (lockdown) would do substantially better in achieving such a decrease than the more moderate forms of social distancing that prevailed for most of March.

As it turns out, the more moderate social distancing techniques in key cases appeared to work sufficiently well to see infection rates peak and begin to decline *before* lockdowns were instituted (Table 2.6). Daily deaths in many countries peaked around the first or second week of April and began to decline. Deaths are a lagging indicator. This means that three weeks before the peak of deaths in April—that is, in the second and third week of March—infections peaked and began to decline. Lockdowns predominately began in the last week of March—well after the decline in the effective reproduction number had kicked in.

Speaking on April 25 2020, Australia's Chief Medical Officer, estimated that the effective reproduction number in the country had reached 1 (the level at which the virus will start to peter out) *before* the country's lockdown restrictions began (Hayne 2020, April 25.)[27] The Norwegian Institute of Public Health on May 5 reported that the nation's R_E level had already fallen to 1.1 *before* Norway's lockdown had been announced (Folkehelseinstituttet 2020, p. 24). On May 22, Camilla Stoltenberg, the Institute's Director General, remarked that "our assessment now....is that we could possibly have achieved the same effects and avoided some of the unfortunate impacts by not locking down, but by instead keeping open but with infection control measures" (Anon 2020c, May 22a). Denmark's Prime Minister Mette Frederiksen announcing her country's lockdown on March 11 said that the measure had been recommended by the nation's *myndighederne*—authorities or agencies. Yet a list of possible measures proposed by the Danish Health Authority on March 10 included few if any lockdown measures (Anon 2020d, May 22b).

In Australia, the state of Queensland introduced a series of lockdown measures including stay-at-home requirements (April 2) and restrictions on "non-essential" businesses (April 9). It gradually lifted these through late April-early July. Looking at the rolling 7-day average of recorded cases in Queensland, the average reproduction rate of virus between March 1 and one week after the lockdown was introduced was 1.1. (Given the one week incubation period of the virus, the effect of any shutdown should not show up in cases for a week). From that one-week post-lockdown marker to July 3, the 7-day average effective reproduction rate was 0.92, barely below the pre-lockdown rate and close to the R_E number (0.95) the week *before* the lockdown was introduced. Queensland's before-and-after R_E numbers strongly suggest that customised and targeted measures rather than the state's broad-band measures would have had as great an impact on the R_E level.

But the COVID state of mind was not simply a political one. It suffused entire societies. Lockdowns were politically popular. They had broad public support—something politicians live for and some at virtually any cost. The shutting down of economies and societies had less to do with practical level-headed measures to reduce the exposure of a population to a virus and more to do with a social mood that had been a long time in development. In 2020 a conjunction of the novel virus and a brittle social atmosphere triggered an unprecedented stampede to close societies to themselves. Numerous currents had shaped this atmosphere. Some belonged to recent decades, others reached back deep into the nineteenth century. All contributed to an overweening sense of social anxiety.

Every individual is calibrated differently. Some deal with fear, including the fear of the unknown, robustly. Others are haunted by fear. Most fit somewhere in-between these poles. As there is individual psychology, there is also mass psychology. Societies from time to time exhibit a collective ego. This is calibrated to be more or less conducive to fear. What was evident in 2020 was the significant number of anxious societies. These concluded that the range of individual prudential responses to COVID-19 was not sufficient in itself. It was not enough for individuals to adhere to public health advisories according to their particular circumstances, level of risk tolerance and personal mechanisms for coping with fear. Instead a collective ego, with a single anxiety setting, had to temporarily take over. Notably in these cases the collective social ego lacked any soulful counterweight. It was earnest and mechanistic to the nth-degree overriding the flexibility and adaptability of the wide spectrum of millions of persons adjusting to exigency in their own adult and level-headed ways.

The collective ego emerged from a mutually reinforcing spiral of public pressure and government response in mid-March 2020. Momentarily it condensed itself into an arrogating social force bent on the epidemiologically impossible project of suppressing the virus. This collective ego crossed all political boundaries. It melded deep anxiety with presumptive confidence in its own power to contain the virus through broad sweeping all-encompassing stay-at-home commands that were at odds with the body of evidence about the virus that had been accumulated between January and mid-March. Social passions subsumed the available dispassionate evidence. Fantasies of "what if" devoured the realities of "what is". Anxiety is a special kind of fear. It is not the fear of a tangible threat. Rather it is the fear of contingency—that is, the fear of what "might be". The COVID moment saw anxious societies briefly spiral down into the fearful anticipation—the dread—of a plague that "might happen". Fear communicates. Panic is communicable. In the COVID episode it spread quickly among all manner of denizens, citizens, householders, journalists, politicians and officials. Visions of pestilence and blight multiplied. But, in the end, the moment of truth was an anti-climax. The plague never came.

Notes

1. The reason for this fell into two categories. One was a prejudice of public health officials against the idea of community immunity, even if the community carriers were low-risk young persons. The second was the fear that education employees—not so much teachers who skew young but ancillary staff who skew older—might be at risk.
2. In a study of Wuhan published in the *New England Journal of Medicine* on January 29, 2020, Li et al. observed that: "It is notable that few of the early cases occurred in children, and almost half the 425 cases were in adults 60 years of age or older, although our case definition specified severe enough illness to require medical attention, which may vary according to the presence of coexisting conditions. Furthermore, children might be less likely to become infected or, if infected, may show milder symptoms, and either of these situations would account for underrepresentation in the confirmed case count. Serosurveys after the first wave of the epidemic would clarify this question."
3. On January 28, the journal *Nature* (Callaway and Cyranoski 2020, January 22) reported: "The WHO last week [*January 21*] published an estimated R0 of 1.4–2.5. Other teams suggest slightly higher values. These estimates are similar to the R0 of SARS during the early stages of the 2002–03 outbreak, and of the novel strain of H1N1 influenza that caused a pandemic in 2009... But researchers caution that R0 estimates come with large uncertainties because of gaps in the data, and the assumptions used to calculate the figure. They also point out that the R0 is a moving target and

that estimates of the figure change over the course of an outbreak." That might have suggested prudential measures to find out more, including testing for the virus and tracking infected persons, but it was hardly reason to panic. Adam Kamradt-Scott, a health-security specialist at the University of Sydney noted that the 1918 influenza outbreak killed 2.5% of those it infected, possibly as many as 50 million people worldwide. The China coronavirus, he told *Nature*, probably would not trigger such an apocalyptic scenario, because it wasn't typically infecting or killing young, healthy people (Lewis 2020, January 31).
4. WHO (World Health Organization) (2020, p. 11). A study of 41 Wuhan hospital patients through to January 2 and published in *The Lancet* on January 24 (Huang et al. 2020) found that 73% of infected patients were men, 32% had underlying diseases, and their median age was 49 years.
5. As of May 1, 2020, there were 27,510 confirmed COVID-related deaths in the UK. Of these 12,526 (45%) were care home residents. Holt and Butcher 2020.
6. The incubation period—the time between exposure to the virus (becoming infected) and the onset of symptoms—is on average is 5–6 days (WHO, 2020, April 2). There are 17.8 days on average from the onset of symptoms to death or discharge from hospital (Verity et al. 2020, March 13).
7. Anon (2020a, March 9).
8. Salje et al. (2020, May 13).
9. * = Greater London boroughs. Dr. Foster, UK Coronavirus Tracker, https://drfoster.com/2020/04/06/uk-coronavirus-tracker/
10. UK Office of National Statistics.
11. Deaths per capita, 21 May 2020: Iceland (29), Taiwan (0.3), Hong Kong (0.5), South Korea (5), Japan (6), Latvia (11), Estonia (48), Sweden (380), Australia (4), United Kingdom (526), Italy (535), Spain (596).
12. The study cited was Kucharski et al. (2020, February 18).
13. Hubei death rate data: China's National Health Commission, Health Commission of Hubei. Zhang et al. 2020 dates the peak of the daily death rate as January 23, 2020.
14. Neil Ferguson was a member of the 17-member expert committee.
15. This is consistent with the experience of the cruise ship, *Diamond Princess*, where the COVID-19 virus spread in a closed and close-contact environment for a month among 3700 passengers and crew. Eventually 19.2% of these were infected.
16. Centers for Disease Control, Pandemic Influenza, Past Pandemics, 1918 Pandemic (H1N1 virus).

17. "[Given] an estimated R0 of 2.4, we predict 81% of the [Great Britain] and US populations would be infected over the course of the epidemic." Ferguson et al. 2020, March 16, p. 6.
18. Avery et al. (2020, April) argue that various social heterogeneities are important in the spread of disease but heterogeneities are not incorporated in standard epidemiological models. They postulate the systematic differences in the patterns of daily life make a single transmission rate for a disease improbable. The strength of network ties to early cases is an example of how social heterogeneity may affect the pace of viral dissemination.
19. A study of 7290 participants and the recorded characteristics of 97,904 contacts.
20. "In China, human-to-human transmission of the COVID-19 virus is largely occurring in families. The Joint Mission received detailed information from the investigation of clusters and some household transmission studies, which are ongoing in a number of Provinces. Among 344 clusters involving 1308 cases (out of a total 1836 cases reported) in Guangdong Province and Sichuan Province, most clusters (78%–85%) have occurred in families. Household transmission studies are currently underway, but preliminary studies ongoing in Guangdong estimate the secondary attack rate in households ranges from 3–10%." WHO, February 16–24, 2020.
21. The scale of spending that this represents was only possible because of low interest rates on bonds.
22. UK Office of National Statistics, Number of deaths registered by week, England and Wales, 28 December 2019 to 8 May 2020.
23. Employment in the US health sector fell by 42,000 jobs in March 2020 (2.3%).
24. Docherty et al. (2020, April 28). The researchers examined data through to April 22 2020.
25. A letter-submission to the South Africa President by the actuaries Nick Hudson and Peter Castleden estimated that South Africa's lockdown would cause a loss of life at least 29 times greater than the loss of life it stood to prevent. The actuaries looked at the aggregate years of life lost (YLL) from two impacts: the impact of COVID-19 overburdening of the South African health system and the impact of economic contraction stemming from COVID-19. The authors assumed a 10–15% decline in GDP in 2020 and a 10–15% unemployment rate. They note that, after 2008, South African employment took five years to fully recover and United States and Euro Area employment took six years. The bottom half of skill and pay grade occupations were the most affected and the slowest to recover. Actuaries use five socio-economic classes to determine relative mortality (life span years) for pricing life insurance. The letter-submission expected

that, with mass employment, 10% of the population would experience the equivalent a drop of one level in socio-economic class for a period of ten years—resulting in a substantial number of years of life lost. Hudson and Castleden (2020, May 5).
26. Of concern were the number of deaths resulting from undiagnosed serious illnesses due to the health industry focus on COVID-19 and the pattern of patients avoiding medical and hospital waiting rooms for fear of being exposed to the virus.
27. Based on a rolling five-day average of new cases reported, the virus' effective reproduction rate reached a peak of 1.39 in Australia on March 12 well before the country's shutdown. Between March 29 and April 24—through Australia's shutdown—the effective reproduction rate varied between 0.99 and 1.11. Cases (unlike deaths) are an imprecise measure of reality—for many cases are not detected. Nonetheless the data indicated a clear trend and approximated what happened.

REFERENCES

Anon. (2020a, March 9). Hospitals told to prepare for bed shortage at peak of virus outbreak. *The Asahi Shimbun.*
Anon. (2020b, May 20). Here's what Sweden's first coronavirus antibody tests tell us. *The Local.*
Anon. (2020c, May 22a). Norway 'could have controlled infection without lockdown': health chief. *The Local.*
Anon. (2020d, May 22b). Danish PM 'falsely claimed health agencies backed lockdown'. *The Local.*
Avery, C. et al. (2020, April). Policy Implications of Models of the Spread of Coronavirus: Perspectives and Opportunities for Economists. *NBER Working Paper Series*, Working Paper 27007.
Bakker, J. (2020, April 9). Lives at risk due to 50% drop in heart attack A&E attendances. *BHF British Heart Foundation.*
Booth, R. (2020, May 20). MPs hear why Hong Kong had no Covid-19 care home deaths. *The Guardian.*
Callaway, E. & Cyranoski, D. (2020, January 22). China coronavirus: Six questions scientists are asking. *Nature.*
Campbell, D. & Mason, R. (2020, May 4). London NHS Nightingale hospital will shut next week. *The Guardian.*
Cheng, H-Y. et al. (2020, May 1). Contact Tracing Assessment of COVID-19 Transmission Dynamics in Taiwan and Risk at Different Exposure Periods Before and After Symptom Onset. *JAMA Internal Medicine.*
Clun, R. (2020, May 9). Don't kiss your mum on Mother's Day, NSW Health Minister says. *Sydney Morning Herald.*

Coombs, B. (2020, April 29). Plunge in health-care spending a big reason US economy sank in first quarter. *CNBC*.
Docherty, K.F. et al. (2020, April 28). Deaths from Covid-19: Who are the forgotten victims? *medRxiv* preprint.
Folkehelseinstituttet. (2020, May 5). *Covid-19-epidemien: kunnskap, situasjon, prognose, risiko og respons i Norge etter uke 18*.
Gardner, J.M. et al. (2020, April 15). *Intervention strategies against COVID-19 and their estimated impact on Swedish healthcare capacity*. medRxiv preprint. https://doi.org/10.1101/2020.04.11.20062133
Ferguson, N. et al. (2020, March 16). *Impact of non-pharmaceutical interventions (NPIs) to reduce COVID-19 mortality and healthcare demand*.
Ghinai, I. et al. (2020, March 13). First known person-to-person transmission of severe acute respiratory syndrome coronavirus 2 (SARS-CoV-2) in the USA. *The Lancet* 395: 1137-1144, March 13, 2020. https://doi.org/10.1016/S0140-6736(20)30607-3
Gomes, M.G.M. et al. (2020, May 2). Individual variation in susceptibility or exposure to SARS-CoV-2 lowers the herd immunity threshold. *medRxiv* preprint. https://doi.org/10.1101/2020.04.27.20081893
Grey, S. & Macaskill, A. (2020, May 5). In shielding its hospitals from COVID-19, Britain left many of the weakest exposed. *Reuters*.
Grifoni, A. et al. (2020, May 7 accepted). Targets of T cell responses to SARS-CoV-2 coronavirus in humans with COVID-19 disease and unexposed individuals. Cell. https://doi.org/10.1016/j.cell.2020.05.015
Hayne, J. (2020, April 25). Coronavirus 'nowcasting' modelling shows Australian case numbers continue to fall. *ABC News* [Australia].
Holt, A. & Butcher, B. (2020, May 15). Coronavirus deaths: How big is the epidemic in care homes? *BBC News*.
Huang, C. et al. (2020, January 24). Clinical features of patients infected with 2019 novel coronavirus in Wuhan, China. *The Lancet*. https://doi.org/10.1016/S0140-6736(20)30183-5
Hudson, N. & Castleden, P. (2020, May 5). Lockdown is a humanitarian disaster to dwarf COVID-19. *PANDA Pandemic Data Analysis*, a letter to President Cyril Ramaphosa, South African President.
IMF (International Monetary Fund). (2020, April). *World Economic Outlook*.
Kucharski A.J. et al. (2020, February 18). Early dynamics of transmission and control of COVID-19: a mathematical modelling study. *medRxiv* preprint. https://doi.org/10.1016/S1473-3099(20)30144-4
Lai, A. et al. (2020, April 28). Estimating excess mortality in people with cancer and multimorbidity in the COVID-19 emergency. preprint *Research Gate*.

Leclerc, Q.J. et al. (2020, June 5). What settings have been linked to SARS-CoV-2 transmission clusters?. *Wellcome Open Research* 5:83.Lewis, D. (2020, January 31). Coronavirus outbreak: what's next? *Nature*, January 31.

Li, Q. et al. (2020, January 29). Early Transmission Dynamics in Wuhan, China, of Novel Coronavirus–Infected Pneumonia. *The New England Journal of Medicine*. https://doi.org/10.1056/NEJMoa2001316

Long, Q-X. et al. (2020, April 29). Antibody responses to SARS-CoV-2 in patients with COVID-19. *Nature Medicine*. https://doi.org/10.1038/s41591-020-0897-1

López, C. (2020, May 13). Sólo 2,3 millones de españoles se han infectado del coronavirus. *Lavanguardia*.

Lynch, L. (2020, April 30). Jeannette Young: who is the woman leading Queensland's fight against COVID-19? *Brisbane Times*.

Mathews, A.W. (2020a, March 26). New York Mandates Nursing Homes Take Covid-19 Patients Discharged From Hospitals. *The Wall Street Journal*.

Mathews, A.W. (2020b, May 14). New York Sent Recovering Coronavirus Patients to Nursing Homes: 'It Was a Fatal Error'. *The Wall Street Journal*.

Mossong, J. et al. (2020, March 28). Social Contacts and Mixing Patterns Relevant to the Spread of Infectious Diseases. *PLOS Medicine*.

NCIRS National Centre for Immunisation Research and Surveillance and NSW Government Health. (2020, April 26). *COVID-19 in schools – the experience in NSW*.

Paavola, A. (2020, April 9). 261 hospitals furloughing workers in response to COVID-19 2020. *Becker's Hospital CFO Report*.

SAGE (Scientific Advisory Group for Emergencies) Committee (2020). *Minutes*, UK Government. Minutes for January 22, January 28, February 3, February 4, February 11, February 13, February 20, February 25, March 3, March 5, March 10, March 13, March 16, March 18, March 23. https://www.gov.uk/government/news/government-publishes-sage-minutes

Salje, H. et al. (2020, May 13). Estimating the burden of SARS-CoV-2 in France. *Science*.

Segal, S. & Gerstel, D. (2020, April 30). Breaking down the G20 Covid-19 Fiscal Response 2020. *Center for Strategic and International Studies*.

Verity, R. et al. (2020, March 13). Estimates of the severity of coronavirus disease 2019: a model-based analysis. *medRxiv* preprint. https://doi.org/10.1101/2020.03.09.20033357

West, D. (2020, April 14). NHS hospitals have four times more empty beds than normal. *HSJ*.

WHO (World Health Organization). (2020, April 2). *Coronavirus disease 2019 (COVID-19) Situation Report – 73*.

Zhang, Z. et al. (2020, April 26). Wuhan and Hubei COVID-19 mortality analysis reveals the critical role of timely supply of medical resources. *Journal of Infection*, in press.

Zhu, Y. et al. (2020, March 30). Children are unlikely to have been the primary source of household SARS-CoV-2 infections. *medRxiv* preprint. https://doi.org/10.1101/2020.03.26.20044826

CHAPTER 3

Social Mood

Abstract The chapter explores the background social thinking that shaped government and public responses to COVID-19. Various ideologies, social moods and belief systems are discussed. Prevailing attitudes to risk, control, government efficacy, human agency, and human freedom are considered. The chapter details how ideas of planning, emergency and calamity, feelings of fear, pessimism and anxiety, and uneasy attitudes to death, human finitude and the future shaped responses to COVID-19.

Keywords Anxiety • Fear • Balance • Freedom • Catastrophism • Futurism • Heroism • Liberalism • Limits • Finitude • Mass events • Realism • Objectivity • Romanticism • Statism • Rationalism • Media • Self-certitude • Exogenous shocks • Stoicism

Public opinion and Mental Contagion
1957–58 saw the spread of the "Asian" influenza (H2N2 virus) epidemic. An estimated 116,000 persons in the United States died from causes related to the virus.[1] That is, 674 per million population. In 1968, the "Hong Kong" influenza (H3N2 virus) epidemic was connected to around 100,000 deaths in the US. That is, 500 deaths per million. As of late May 2020, the United States (one of the globe's more severely affected nations) was tracking to match the estimated virus-related death toll from the

© The Author(s) 2020
P. Murphy, *COVID-19*,
https://doi.org/10.1007/978-981-15-7514-3_3

1957–58 flu.[2] Yet the reaction of governments and publics worldwide to COVID-19 (America included) proved by an order of magnitude to be much more obsessive and zealous than during the pandemics of 1957–58 and 1968. No shutdown of societies or economies occurred in either 1958 or 1968.

What happened in late March and April 2020 was a form of collective hysteria about a serious yet not catastrophic public health matter. Governments and publics both panicked. Hysteria is a kind of mental contagion. Once it is set running, it overwhelms all other considerations for a time. Then as swiftly it recedes. At its height it tolerates no opposition. It cannot be questioned. It is as infectious as a viral pathogen. But like viruses its effective reproduction number at some point begins to decline. The social body forms anti-bodies to the mental virus. Calm is restored.

Public opinion routinely operates much like a viral contagion. Have you ever wondered why political and social issues suddenly appear out of nowhere, rise swiftly in public notice for a period of time and then plateau until the amount of attention paid to them declines, often sharply? This is because public opinion is communicable—that is, it is contagious. Certain issues transmit rapidly from one person to another. These issues have brief periods of exponential growth. That is, in each case, a brief take-off moment. Then growth of interest in the issue slows but still continues to grow at a fair pace until it plateaus and the process is reversed. An issue that happens to be pervasive at one point in time, two years later may barely be remembered.

When it is pervasive an issue generates more noise than information. It is often the case that what appears to be evidence introduced to promote one or other side of an issue turns out to be a talking point. This is a way of increasing the communicability of the issue but to the detriment of its substance or meaning. Media—be it newspapers, broadcasters or social media—on the whole exhibited a poor understanding of COVID-19 evidence. A day's spike in cases or deaths was confused with a trend. The cherry-picking of the worst day's data was extrapolated on a linear basis into the future. Virus growth was routinely interpreted as though it was an unbending line projected in one direction rather than a bell-curve. Case fatalities were confused with infection fatalities. Asymptomatic persons were excluded when calculating infection fatality rates. If case numbers increased because of expanded testing, the assumption was made that things were getting worse while in fact the number of cases hadn't changed—just more of them were being discovered. In reality no more deaths would occur as a result of more cases being uncovered and registered.

As a general rule, headlines gravitated to the worst scenarios. So did the responses of the larger majority of newspaper readers and social media followers. This is a common feature of public opinion: negative information bias. Good news does not sell. Human beings are attracted to images of disaster and doom. Through March, April and May 2020, media of all kinds functioned primarily as an echo chamber. The chamber repeated official clichés. The most prominent of these was the phrase "flatten the curve" the use of which exploded in mid-March. As it turned out no national COVID curve was ever flattened. Nation by nation the curve either peaked steeply or its top was rounded. A flattened curve would have been drawn out for many months until it finally tapered off. We saw no example of that. Just as quickly as it entered national lexicons, the phrase "flatten the curve" disappeared, almost overnight.

Mentalities, Politics, Beliefs
Why in March, April and May 2020 did the COVID-19 issue transmit virally for a time—virtually precluding all other discussion of public issues? What in this case put the contagion into public opinion and set it running feverishly? No one factor explains this. On the contrary numerous factors were in play. These came together like a huge spark igniting public opinion and causing the COVID-19 issue to spread like wild-fire among opinion makers, executive governments, politicians, the media and the public at large. Among the factors that coalesced in the COVID moment were the following:

3.1 MENTALITIES

3.1.1 Catastrophism

For decades over-wrought and apocalyptic scenarios have periodically gripped the world—be they about environmental calamity, computer cataclysms, nuclear accidents, terrorism and food poisoning. The apocalypse is an old religious idea. It originally meant a struggle of good against an evil that lays waste to world. The struggle is painful and destructive. The world ends. But the end-times is a precursor of a world of divine beatitude in union with God. In secular modernity the idea of the apocalypse leading to some kind of divine exaltation or blessed state disappeared. However the catastrophic nature of the idea of the apocalypse was retained. Catastrophism and end-of-the world scenarios appear remarkably often in arguments about public policy. They are the direct antithesis of prudential arguments.

Prudence relies on calm and composure in contrast to feelings of impending doom. The prudential mentality is one that avoids thinking in terms of extremes, be it exaltation or convulsion. Prudence is closely related to the epistemologies of the observer or the spectator. These focus on the observation of reality rather than over-heated projections of what "might" happen. Just as stock markets from time to time exhibit irrational exuberance in their behaviour so projections of the future at times exhibit irrational exaggerations ["sublimities"]. Irrational exaggerations come in many forms including the anti-scientific and the nominally scientific. They all involve to some degree the hallucinatory imagining of a lurid future.

3.1.2 *Alarmism*

Secular apocalyptic scenarios are typically built on predictions of widespread harm and destruction. These predictions are matched by various forms of psychological hyper-sensitivity. The prominence of anxiety and depression in the mass psychology of the last century seeded the ground for alarmism. Alarmism is a kind of communicable nervousness. It is typically triggered in response to predictions of apocalyptic social harm. Predictions of disaster and alarmed responses to such predictions feed off each other. A downward spiral occurs. Forecasts of disaster beget anxious responses that beget statements of alarm that beget further, even more intense disaster forecasts. The cycle goes on and on until it reaches a pitch of hysterical intensity and then subsides.

3.1.3 *Pessimism*

Then there is the legacy of 2008. The world economy recovered in three years after the Global Financial Crisis of 2008. But the legacy of cognitive and emotional despair caused by the shock of that event, the most serious downturn since the Great Depression, left significant parts of populations in the major economies with a mental outlook dominated by pessimistic, hyperbolic, and anxious thoughts. In those parts of society that were most deeply affected by 2008, stress coping mechanisms were impaired by the initial deep shock and the after-waves of the downturn. The number and extent of anxious social contagions increased. The characteristic medium of the 2010s—social media—facilitated and in many respects exemplified this process of moral contagion. However it was not alone. Media in general through the 2010s echoed the pessimism, hyperbole and anxiety of the post-2008 era.

3.1.4 Futurism

In principle modelling is a way of predicting the course of novel mass events. If a shock event occurs there is an understandable desire to know what the future holds. From oracles and prophecies to social forecasting and economic predictions, that desire has remained the same over millennia. The future is made up of predictable routine events and surprising shocks. The sun rises in the morning and the stock market unexpectedly crashes. Predicting routine events—like the daily weather—is modestly successful. The ability to predict surprises—exceptional events that startle and stun—is rare. When events daze, confuse and scare people on a large scale, it is a sign that the future has entered unknown territory. Human beings have a strong desire to know the unknowable—and it is understandable that they will try to do that. But the very nature of what makes shock-wave events so startling is that they are driven by an uncertain mix of multiple causes that interact in ways that follow no well-established and empirically mapped routine or pattern. This makes the modelling of mass shock events effectively often little more reliable than the pronouncements of oracles and prophets.

3.1.5 Realism

Mass events are governed by the patterns of big numbers—fractals, ratios, bell curves, averages, coefficients, clusters, per capita figures and the like. Empirical observation allows us to establish what patterns are at play in the midst of mass events. Observational knowledge usually does not allow us to control or suppress mass events. But typically mass events can be gradually mitigated by virtue of adaptive behaviour. Even when explicit knowledge of the underlying pattern behaviour of shock events does not exist, human beings nevertheless are good at adapting to these events even if they are poor at controlling them. Realism is the acceptance of this along with the acceptance that reality (in the case of large-scale jolting events) cannot be usefully modelled, though close observation of empirical reality as it twists and turns can provide useful knowledge about these events. The realist is sceptical of sooth-saying forecasting.

While mass events are imprinted in the consciousness of modern persons, most individuals do not like big numbers. Such numbers appear to be—and in truth are—abstractions. To say that 600,000 persons die annually in Britain and that any reasonable estimate of COVID-19 deaths will be a modest-to-moderate portion of that number is lost on populations that wish everything to be personalised and concretised. But what makes modern societies tick is their scale and (with that scale) the patterns of large numbers. Modern populations are more often drawn to magical realism than they are to metrical realism. They prefer banging on a drum to the quiet ticking of the metronome. Some of the effects of mass events can be seen. They are visible to the eye. They happen in the here and now. Other effects are not visible because they are delayed. They do not appear for months, years or decades. The unseen effects of mass events are as important—if not more important—than the immediate visible effects of those events. But the distinction between the visible and the invisible also is an abstraction, and, as such, is at odds with the mind-set of the personality who is interested only in concrete specifics in the here-and-now. The same tension between the abstract and the concrete repeats itself in politics between the retail politician who is sensitive to the voter who thinks in terms of visible tangibles and the metrical realist who is used to balancing the present and the future, costs and benefits, and inputs and outcomes.

3.1.6 Rationalism

The policy sciences are divided between metrical realists and rationalists. Reason is the faculty that we have for finding the right means to deliver the ends we want. Rationalists deploy the faculty of reason in a particular way. They typically isolate or prioritize *one* end. That favoured end excludes or else significantly de-prioritizes other ends. In the mind of the rationalist, reason is not a faculty in the service of several ends but rather in the service of *the* end. In the COVID case, *the* end is to reduce or eliminate the death toll from the virus. Rationalism always has a noble end. Its nobility though is one-eyed. *The* end in this case justifies not just the means used but crucially it excludes other competing ends. Rationalism is mono-manic. Or perhaps another way to put it: rationalism is obsessive. And curiously, as a consequence, rationalism is irrational. It is reason elevated to the point of irrationality. It is the irrational side of reason. Thus the policy rationalist can say: forget anything but COVID deaths. Forget ancillary deaths from reduced hospital referrals or waiting-room avoidance. Forget deaths from despair. Forget economic gutting. Instead, the only thing that matters are COVID deaths. Focus on those alone.

3.1.7 Pluralism

The metrical realist's response to the rationalist is that inherently there is a pluralism of goods and not just one good only. A balance or an equilibrium has to be struck between competing goods. This is part of what we call prudence or good judgment. Good policy judgment means being able to trade off the needs of one value against that of another value, one benefit against another benefit, one cost against another cost. This requires a certain shrewdness in working out how best to achieve that. It needs a sharp minds-eye to see the various goods at stake in any given decision. The pluralist and the rationalist necessarily find themselves at loggerheads. For the rationalist there is only one direction to go in. There can be no compromise, no weighing up of competing considerations, and no stopping. For the pluralist, the overriding mentality is quantum in nature: there are competing goods and those goods have to be brought together in a way that resembles quantum super-positioning.

3.1.8 Moralism

We tend to think of public opinion as a space in which conflicting opinions clash and argue. To an extent this is true. But more often public opinion is not a realm of opinions (plural) but rather an opinion (singular) that functions in effect as an external authority in the way that the state for example functions as an external authority.[3] Public opinion singular tends to be aggressive and intimidating. It does not like dissent or disagreement or being called into question. It is "right", a supreme social repository of justified true belief. Its rightness—its validity—rests on its being widely held. This in turn supports all manner of over-bearing and heated insistence that it is "right". Anger, vehemence, passion, enthusiasm, superciliousness, scorn and disdain are mobilised in support of public opinion in the singular as defences against its very "obviousness" being called into question.

Public opinion in the singular is the externalisation (as a social authority) of internal self-certitude. It is self-certitude projected as a social force. It is not a very tolerant or forgiving external authority. Alexis de Tocqueville in the 1830s noted its propensity to despotism—specifically a kind of democratic despotism. Its lack of tolerance stems from the nature of its source in self-certitude. Self-certitude is the internal mechanism—part cognition, part emotion—that allows persons to think that they are "right" and "certain" about a matter with little or no evidence that that is so. It is not intuition, instinct or gut feeling but rather an internal feeling of certainty that reassures the person that their course of action is "correct". It is an emotional-cognitive response to uncertainty or contingency, which rapidly asserts a kind of felt certainty in the absence of any real evidence for the belief. "I *feel* I am right." On a grand social level, self-certainty externalized as public opinion (singular) gives individuals the warrant to make insistent, loud, moralising statements and gestures that preclude discussion, criticism or reflection on the grounds that measure A is "correct" or "self-evident" without any need for discussion, criticism or reflection. Governments mirror the authority of public opinion in the singular with their own reluctance having adopted a course of action ever to admit they were wrong. Even about tiny things, governments having made a decision will rarely if ever acknowledge that it was the wrong course of action.

3.2 Politics

The COVID moment was not a good time for metrical realists. The combination of rationalism, pessimism, alarmism and catastrophism shoved them to one side. The gale force of COVID's policy rattle and bluster was amplified by the resurgence of a phalanx of political trends, many of them long latent in the invisible repository of modern political thought. No idea dies, it seems. It just slumbers away till its time comes again. The COVID moment coalesced strands of thinking derived from socialism's planning state, liberalism's regulatory state, rationalism's bureaucratic state, communism's command-state, and constitutionalism's state of exception (the constitutional emergency state). Traces of all of these played a part in the world's COVID lockdown moment.

3.2.1 Romanticism

The lockdown strategy originated in Communist China. It resembled in many respects Johann Fichte's influential idea of a closed commercial economy. German Romanticism's powerful fantasy-image of a closed economy and society minutely regulated by the state has long had a following in various guises and forms. In the COVID moment this dream was realized on a world scale for a month. Persons were locked-down in their houses. Freedom of movement, that most fundamental of liberties, was suspended. Nations banned air travel. "Inessential" commerce was forbidden while "essential" commerce was permitted. Romanticism is the source of the modern autarchic vision of a shuttered society immune from exogenous impacts. Suspending the freedom of movement was reminiscent of totalitarian societies, the step-children of Romanticism. That China inaugurated the lockdown policy was unsurprising. That the liberal-democracies followed suit was surprising. That Sweden, well-known for its large state, was one of the few democracies that refused to become temporarily an illiberal carceral society was perhaps most surprising of all.

3.2.2 Asceticism

"Inessential" commerce is a recurring political theme that we hear from time to time. On this view, human beings possess "real needs" and "false needs". Consumption, or a large part of it, is one of the "false needs". Driven by false needs, we consume what is "inessential". We are seduced by all manner of indulgence, frippery and inauthenticity. We commit unnecessary or destructive expenditures of time, money, resources and energy. If only the world was frugal. From this vantage-point, the real disease of the world is consumerism. Lockdowns are good because they prefigure a world that consumes less and uses less. The promise of shutdowns is that the ascetic priests—the experts in other persons' abstemiousness and the state managers of social prohibitions—one day will oversee a society where abstinent and self-denying behaviour is the norm and everything is meticulously rationed by those who administer a closed commercial state.

3.2.3 Organic Solidarity

Even socialism, or at least one of its numerous off-spring, momentarily returned in the COVID moment: in the form of the resurrection of Emile Durkheim's image of a state-orchestrated organic solidarity. For a few weeks globally the world of shutdown turned togetherness (social solidarity) into a function of emergency executive action that directed human beings to achieve togetherness through physical separation. In the case of Durkheim's mechanical solidarity—the glue of archaic societies—each part of society is more or less the same as all other parts—making togetherness a simple function of social being. In the case of modern societies, which are highly differentiated, and in a lockdown are physically differentiated, togetherness (solidarity) occurs in and through the state. By limiting interaction outside the home, governments did something that was reminiscent of the atomisation of totalitarian societies but with two important qualifications. The stay-at-home orders were a temporary not a permanent condition. And while social interaction outside the household decreased dramatically, virtual interaction beyond the household increased and was not regulated. Nonetheless the state for a discrete period of time became at least society's most effective and prominent social bond—generating thereby a high degree of interest in the statements and symbols of prime ministers and health officials. The degree to which this temporary housebound society was disconnected from its usual physical peer networks was the degree to which the state became the connector of the social atoms.

3.2.4 The Emergency State

In the COVID moment, Durkheim's image of organic solidarity was combined with and effectively mediated by Carl Schmitt's model of the emergency state. In an emergency, the state can use its constitutional powers to rule by decree or instruction. A constitutional state of emergency is a form of temporary, that is to say, exceptional authority. The state is authorized to rule for a period of time through the medium of directions rather than laws. This temporary form of power exists for the explicit purpose of combatting an emergency. It is based on the ancient Roman model of the constitutional dictator. In the case of COVID-19 the emergency was a public health emergency with apocalyptic connotations that tapped into a well-spring of public and government alarmism that had developed over decades. The justification for the emergency authority was to control the virus and thereby save lives.

3.2.5 The Planned State

The idea that the state could control a virus is consistent with the essential nature or make-up of the state. At its core, the state is an agency of control. That is, in normal circumstances, it establishes parameters of human behaviour ranging from laws to instructions. In the COVID moment, governments issued copious instructions from "wash your hands" to "stay at home". Mass shock events can be controlled to a degree. But—and this is the dilemma, indeed the conundrum—only ever to a degree. How far does control go before it becomes futile or even counter-productive? For the rationalist control can never go far enough.

The COVID moment was replete with rationalist methods: government stages, steps, schedules, and levels abounded. Each implied a plan. These plans were based on models of the virus' future behaviour. This modelling was reminiscent of the old Communist idea of a centrally-planned economy. Its flaw was the same as its predecessor. Planners can never have sufficient knowledge of all the innumerable working parts of an economy, so they can never actually plan its development so that plan and reality coincide. Similarly, modellers can never possess sufficient knowledge of all the factors that determine the dissemination and mitigation of a virus and the way these multiple factors interact—speeding and impeding the spread of the virus. This is a problem of the limits of human knowledge—which also means the limits of the state's ability to plan and thus control any outcome. Those limits as they applied to economic plans were widely understood by the 1970s. Yet bad ideas persist in new forms. So that even after the demise of various twentieth-century ideologies of planning—which once were commonplace—the desire to plan has remained with us because we have a strong desire to control the future. Simply having this desire though does not make either models or plans effective. The ability to control either the natural or social environment, or a mix of both in the case of pandemics, is inherently limited. Control—or rather attempts at it—can have serious negative unintended consequences. Yet the inclination of the planner is not to observe and (surgically) respond to mass events but rather to foresee them and in foretelling those events (prophetically) decide how to intervene and control them.

3.2.6 Freedom

Freedom is crucial to civil societies. But COVID can't be construed simply as a civil liberties issue, even though governments did in essence lock up populations for a month or more in their own homes. The COVID episode in interesting ways posed the question of the antinomy of freedom. What is most powerful socially are concepts that have a nexus with their opposites. So it is with freedom and discipline. We admire free societies. But we also admire societies that are disciplined and that don't fritter away freedom in indulgent behaviour. Can one be free *and* disciplined? That requires the bridging concept of responsibility. A responsible person is a free person who is sufficiently disciplined not to cause others foreseeable harm. Social distancing is a behavioural discipline that a free but responsible person can engage in, in order to mitigate the COVID virus.

Responsibility is the resolution of the antinomy of freedom and discipline. When states replace the self-responsibility of their populations with regulatory directives and paternalistic stay-at-home orders they are violating the principles of a free society just as free but undisciplined actions also undermine the foundations of a free society. Modern state paternalism is the fruit of romantic socialism. Modern wilful freedom is the fruit of romantic expressivism. Their philosophical source is the same even if their demeanour is different. In the COVID moment, the free and responsible person got squashed between a rush to embrace the paternal state and to paint sceptics of lockdowns as partisans of wilful freedom. Walking solo in a national park or playing a solo round of golf became for a brief time acts of wilful freedom and dangerous affronts to a paternal state whose business it was to "look after" all its "children" not least the population of adults who it had decided, as a matter of care, were incapable of self-responsibility. Yet in many states (not all) that paternalism failed in the case where it was most justified—in the case of nursing homes, filled with persons who cannot look after themselves who were known from early reporting of COVID to be the most vulnerable to its pathogen. Rather than targeted proportionality that matched the paternal state with the most vulnerable persons, states chose to infantilize whole populations of adults at low risk rather than ask them to exercise responsible freedom.

3.3 Beliefs

3.3.1 Explanatory Beliefs

Beliefs (among other things) provide explanations of why mass events happen. Modern societies routinely feel the shock effects of such events. Economic booms and recessions, rates of suicide and mortality, the relative prevalence of contentment and worry, patterns of social intimacy and distance like seasonal illnesses and pandemics all occur on a mass scale. Explanatory beliefs provide individuals with reasons "why" a mass event occurs. Like personal assumptions and expectations, beliefs tend to be forms of self-certitude. They provide psychological certainty in the face of society's contingencies and especially in the face of threatening contingencies. However, most explanatory beliefs are wrong. Self-certitude, while it is comforting, is not a source of reliable knowledge.

In the COVID moment, false explanations proliferated. They did so among citizens, publics, governments, politicians, officials, academics, journalists and commentators. Explanatory beliefs are frequently false because they tend to focus on a single cause for a given phenomenon and will do so without any substantial evidence—or any evidence at all—that the reputed cause is actually causative. In contrast most mass social events, like the impact of COVID, have multiple causes. They don't lend themselves to "easy" explanations. Yet comfort-explanations need to be simple. Part of their simplicity is that they can be believed irrespective of any plausible or contrary evidence. It might be comforting to believe conspiracy theories or claims of panaceas and magical remedies or even more plausible-sounding speculations (e.g. that the virus attack rate was highest in very dense cities). But like most of the rampant COVID explanations, these claims were based on no real supporting empirical evidence or effective observation or else, in the case of conspiracy theories, on a thicket of made-up evidence.

3.3.2 Consolatory Beliefs

The will to believe is powerful. In no small part this is because persons seek consolation and reassurance in difficult times. That's a normal human response to bad events. Belief induces certainty. Belief is a cognitive feeling—really in fact more feeling than cognition. If we believe X (no matter how unrealistic it might be), then we become more confident that Y will occur. If we believe that an unproven or quack remedy can "treat" the virus, we become more confident that a patient who is seriously ill with the virus will have a therapeutic treatment that will mean they won't end up in an ICU with a low probability of surviving. Beliefs are emotionally reassuring that the things we fear or about which we are anxious will not happen or will be overcome.

3.3.3 Heroism

During the COVID episode, doctors and nurses were thought of as being on the "front line", battling an overwhelming disease. The nation was fighting a virtual Blitz. The archaic image of the warrior-hero was reformulated for a procedural and institutional world as the emergency services or hospital hero. These were the ones, in the midst of a shuttered world, who answered the call, left home every day to travel to a place of horror in order to do battle with a menacing evil and slay the evil. The difficulty for public policy was to separate consolatory belief, perfectly understandable in a time suffused by the fear of death, with the hard cold evidence of the actual demands on hospitals, the fear of going to hospitals because of COVID scares, the methods of virus transmission, and the cohorts at risk from death.

Modern societies are procedural in spirit in the same way that traditional societies were habitual in spirit. Neither the rules of institutions nor the ingrained habits of a society are very inspiring. From them societies derive their regularity. Rules and habits are recipes for action. They can in varying degrees be functional or dysfunctional. However in all degrees they are bland and unexciting. No one is filled with exhilaration when they follow rules or customs. That's the nature of social life. It means though that many people have an unsatisfied taste for a heroic "something" that is outside the normal. In the contemporary era we see the massive consumption of super-hero movies. Visualizing the imaginary hero in some kind of extreme situation is a release from routine, be it the quotidian routines bound up with the cycles of work and life, or the procedural rule-following of modern organizations and institutions.

COVID offered persons unconsciously a heroic moment—either by identification with the imagined extremes of emergency conditions or else identification with the presumptive heroism of emergency service and hospital workers, applauded for valour exhibited in fulfilling a high purpose, like knights fighting (in this case) the plague. Whether in many cases the shifts of these workers were less routine or more stressed or more dangerous than the two months of a very bad flu season is an impolitic question to ask, even insensitive, when the will to believe in a compensatory heroism is very strong. Everyone likes that some kind of exceptional bravery may be attributed to a group. In such cases what is important is myth not reality. Myths release energies and motivate life. They are not descriptive or explanatory but rather inspiring and rousing. Story-telling and the hero narrative are deeply encoded in the human psyche. This is part of who we are. But the difficulty is that mass events, which have become increasingly prominent in modern societies, both in a positive and negative way, do not lend themselves to narrative explanations nor to stories of heroes and sacrificial individuals.

Social science once would have provided non-narrative explanations for mass social events. But it was mostly silent during the COVID moment. It had little to say on the matter. But whether charismatic myths and stories or belief in the authority of science can replace it is an open question. As far as the myth of the super-hero is concerned, the desire of persons to be released from routine life—be it everyday life or institutional life—even if only momentarily is understandable. But whether the charisma of the super-man is sufficient to justify, or even partly justify, a shutdown of an economy or a society is another matter altogether.

3.3.4 *The Fear of Death*

As the philosopher Thomas Hobbes observed in the seventeenth century, the fear of death is a building block for the modern state. It is the cement that binds government and public together in the modern (Hobbesian) social contract. It motivates a mix of government intervention and protection. This assumes—and promises—that the sovereign (today: executive government) has compelling powers including emergency powers that are built on a responsibility for and a power over life and death. The populations of panicking nations look to the state for reassurance and action. April 2020 saw a brief moment of "epidemiarchy". Public health officials, whom the public usually ignore, became celebrities in the public spotlight. Democratic states followed the model of authoritarian China and locked down their societies and economies. So much so that, for a time, this was reminiscent of the feudal peasant tied to the soil.

China's Communist Party routinely restricts the freedom of movement of its population. How could this happen in liberal democracies, where the freedom of movement is one of the basic assumptions and rights? The answer is the fear of death. Hobbes supposed that warfare among human tribes and societies—and the ensuing fear of death—would cause individuals to agree to obey a sovereign power that in return would protect them.

Fear of viral death saw a ready surrender of liberal freedoms in the name of protection and the promise of state intervention to control the virus. How well-founded the fear was is debatable. But it certainly had the effect of populations, for a time, waiving their normal freedoms for something that much more resembled a momentary despotic state. In part at least this readiness was a consequence of deep ambivalences about the nature and meaning of death in societies that, 350 years on from Hobbes, because of medical science, have conquered most premature deaths and yet which remain curiously uncertain about what this means. If anything the more we have been able to control the onset of death and extend life span, the more fearful we have become about the prospect of death.

3.3.5 *The Fear of Finitude*

Contemporaries are uncomfortable with death. Belief in an after-life has diminished. Yet reconciliation with the fact of mortal finitude and the limits of the "this-worldly existence" has not replaced it. If we neither believe that "death is not the end" nor fully accept that "life is finite" and that death in old-age is a natural limit that gives shape, form and meaning to each life, then anxieties about death are apt to become over-heated and eventually hysterical. Tensions, manifest in public opinion, exist between conceptions of extending life-span, the inherent limits (the finiteness) of life-span, residual ideas about an after-life or re-birth, and models of the heroic medical prolongation of life. Conflicting unreconciled images of immortality, a fulfilled life, an eternal life—and myriad this-worldly and other-worldly promises—haunt social thinking about mortality.

3.3.6 *The Fear of Strangers*

Though atypical, at times stranger interaction has been a model for personal interaction. In the English cultural tradition, this was true both of the Georgian (Jane Austen-style) formalistic and the Victorian inhibited model of behaviour in personal relationships. These fell out of favour in the 1960s. After 1970, the model of uninhibited Romantic-expressive relationships became more common. The health consequences of this first became apparent during the 1980s AIDS epidemic. Romantic-expressive philosophies in a demotic setting are the "touchy-feely" philosophies that emphasise breaking down the tactile and proxemic barriers between people. Authentic human relations are close, "in your face" relationships. Distance is equated with coldness. Proximity is equated with warmth. Touch is an expression of community, the perpetual dream of Romanticism. The underlying intellectual myth or fantasy is the merging of two bodies in one. The hope is to be made whole again, in an expressive oneness, after civilization has divided person from person in the same way allegedly that it has divided humankind from nature and the individual from the state. Romantic-expressive philosophies widely entered the cultural mainstream after the 1960s. They coloured many aspects of mainstream culture including child-rearing practices that teach pre-school children their tacit concepts of proximity and distance. From the romantic radicals of the 1960s core romantic ideas gradually entered into the quotidian mores of the broader society. The consequence was that many people, even if only unconsciously or mimetically, sought an expressive closeness in all manner of human relationships.

In successful societies in modernity the image of the stranger made significant headway. It facilitated pattern-based behaviour in favour of rule-based or command-based behaviour. The former was key to the spread of markets, technologies and publics. But the stranger also has always been a figure of fear and anxiety. Societies have never quite resolved these attractions and repulsions. The distance of the stranger lends life objectivity and calm. But it makes people feel that their fellows are "estranged" from them, insufficiently like them. They feel a gulf of separation that they want to bridge. They want to reach out, touch and somehow fuse with the other person. They feel a need to loosen their inhibitions in doing so. They want to merge with the other person, and feel annoyed and hurt when they are denied the symbols of doing so, be it ever so ordinary as the kiss on the cheek or the hand brushing the face. The more ordinary, the better. For the symbolic merger of bodies in acts of expressive closeness occurs at a micro-social level. It happens all around us. We swim, almost unawares, barely at threshold of consciousness, in a sea of touch and proximity.

Our communitarian brain—our social brain—tells us that risk comes from strangers (the population as a whole) not from intimates. In the COVID case the opposite was true—prolonged contact with persons we know well was the primary medium of transmission of the virus. Hugs, handshakes, kisses, and embraces facilitated the transmission of the disease. Close sustained contact was the problem. But we have thousands of years of the communitarian brain that, in some cases, gives an absolute priority to close contact relationships. In the COVID case this was a pronounced liability both for being infected and for analysing the specific character (channels) by which the infection was communicated. We naturally seek security in those closest to us. But that is not in every case wise.

The space between human beings is emotionally charged. We constantly negotiate it. Fear, anxiety and uncertainty tends to cause us to increase the space separating us from others. If we are wary of others, we step back, even if only ever so slightly. We keep our distance. But paradoxically the shrinking of intimate space is also the by-product of fears and anxieties. We hug a child who is fearful. The act is reassuring. It is a form of emotional sheltering. We seek security by being close to others. But on occasions this is not always prudent. Yet it is difficult to countermand our in-built, tacit social behavioural norms. We feel the space between us rather than think on it or reflect on it.

3.3.7 Emotivism

In the past 50 years, post-1970, the habit of treating acquaintances (e.g. colleagues) as if they were intimates has grown. The annual Christmas party has mutated into the multiple works drinks, BBQs, outings, drinks after work, etc. The office partition gave way to the open-plan office. Social life gravitated to work locations. The latent hostility often encountered in workplaces was offset by a fake sociability marked by kisses on the cheek, back slapping, tight-space pub gatherings, team bonding, and so on. The deeper social drivers of this were post-1968 romantic expressivism and pre-68 forms of ethical emotivism that sought to restrict the distancing effect of social manners. Both were resistant to cognitive objectivism. In both cases, hopes, dreams, fantasies and expectations sought to override facts. One can reasonably disagree about facts. But one can also unreasonably ignore them.

3.3.8 The Death of God

Once it was God, not governments, which had a plan. In the case of God, this was a providential plan. That plan may have been inscrutable to those who suffered yet it provided a reason (viz. God's design) that made sense of that suffering, no matter how undeserved or arbitrary it might have been. God's design however opaque gave that suffering a meaning and made it thereby easier to bear. In a more general way, religion provided an account of not only those things that were within our power to control but also what was outside of human control.

Religion pointed to something greater or larger than humankind. That which was more powerful than ordinary human agency encompassed everything from an abstract depersonalised Deist nature to a wrathful commanding God. In modernity, gradually, human will replaced providence. Science promised (and in part achieved) the prospect that human beings would control nature. Government promised that human beings could control economies and societies by instructions, commands and plans. Providential plans were replaced by organizational plans, necessity by directed free will, and preordination by prediction. The end result of this was the promise of secular redemption. Rather than the individual sinner being saved, the state and its agencies promised to save society even if necessary from itself. In the case of COVID-19 it promised the deliverance of society from the plague. Following the logic of this redemptive politics, the United Kingdom turned its National Health Service (NHS) into a pseudo church. Doctors became "saints"; nurses "angels". The nation at large periodically went about happy clapping the NHS. This was the secular and state equivalent of a charismatic religion—clapping and shouting during religious services, and worshipping with the body and not just the mind.

3.3.9 Stoicism

This is not to say that prediction, free will and administrative plans are fruitless or irrelevant. Calculating the future, choosing what we do and when we do it, and matching means with ends in a methodical fashion are valuable. But so also is the acknowledgement of necessity, which a deep sense of destiny and implacability provides. Not everything in the world is foreseeable. Not everything can be reduced to choices or plans. Not everything can be determined while much in fact can be adapted to as long as we recognize the difference between what can be changed and what cannot be changed. The Stoic formula is: Accept what you cannot change; change what is in your power to change. Many things we experience are not changeable while some are. This Stoic precept applies to governments as much as to publics. Human purposefulness is limited. So too is government capacity to enact its purposes. Governments like individuals are ill-suited to broad spectrum actions that enact change or attempt to realise purposes on a broad macro-scale. Human purposiveness is suited to the small scale and mid-scale. The wider the scope of change the less likely it is to be successful. Successful purposive action is surgical in nature. When opening up the social body it aims to make the smallest incision that will yield the greatest results.

Aftermath

Climbing back down from March, April and May 2020 will be difficult. The government-engineered recessions will leave deep economic and psychological scars world-wide. The enthusiastic emotional investment of publics and governments in lockdowns will leave a legacy of deep ambivalence: guilt for over-reacting combined with denial that an over-reaction occurred. We will see a defiant insistence that lockdowns were "necessary", an uneasy conscience that they were not "necessary", a sense of culpability and contrition at the damaging consequences of lockdowns, and a feeling of being haunted by 2020 as earlier decades were haunted by 2008, 2001 and 1989.

Notes

1. Centres for Disease Control, Pandemic Influenza, Past Pandemics, 1957–1958 Pandemic (H2N2 virus).
2. In some cases a second wave of infection followed the COVID-19 wave in March-May 2020 or perhaps more accurately in the case of Arizona, Texas and Florida in the United States a belated first wave occurred through June and July 2020. The wave pattern of virus outbreaks vary. The SARS virus impacted Hong Kong in one wave between March and May 2003; in Toronto the SARS outbreak occurred in two phases, March to April and May to June with a bottoming out between April 29 and May 11. The Spanish Influenza of 1918–1919 was the most deadly pandemic of the last century. In Australia the Spanish flu occurred in three waves: the first wave in January-February 1919; the second wave in mid-March-April and a third wave in June-July. 15,000 Australians died from the pandemic—3000 per million population. 40% of the population was infected (Defining Moments, ND). The New South Wales government imposed lock-downs through the first and second waves. By the third wave it gave up. In the first and second waves it made masks mandatory (but not on public transport, one of many

policy inconsistencies pointed out by critics) and required libraries, schools, churches, theatres, public halls, and entertainment venues to close. Debates about the wisdom of these measures were eerily similar to debates today. Once the third wave hit the government did not reimpose restrictions, aware of the effect on employment, and the previous unsuccessful attempt to supress the virus. It decided third time round to allow the virus to run its course, saying wisely that "there is a stage at which governmental responsibility for the public health ends" and indicating that the population by that point should have been aware of the gravity of the situation and capable of acting responsibly in the face of that knowledge (Kildea 2020, May 22).

3. An example is the number of videos of serious epidemiologists that YouTube removed from its service during the COVID episode on the grounds that the views put forward by these scientists were inconsistent with the authority of the World Health Organization. Science is this case becomes an authority. In other words it becomes a form of scientism. Science properly speaking is not an authority but rather involves the ability to question and argue on informed and rational grounds. Scientism is a sign of how far science today has moved away from the criterion of falsifiability introduced by the philosopher of science Karl Popper. That is, any credible scientific proposition must be capable of being disproved. If it is right only by virtue of authority, then it is not a scientific proposition. The Chief Executive of Youtube stated that "Anything that would go against World Health Organization recommendations would be a violation of our policy" (News 2020, April 22).

REFERENCES

Defining Moments. (ND). 1919: Influenza pandemic reaches Australia. *National Museum of Australia.*

Kildea, J. (2020, May 22). Lockdowns, second waves and burn outs. Spanish flu's clues about how coronavirus might play out in Australia. *The Conversation.*

News (2020, April 22). Coronavirus: YouTube bans 'medically unsubstantiated' content. *BBC.*

AFTERWORD

October 10, 2020. This book was written in May 2020. It was concerned with events principally in March through May. Those events continued after that. However in the main they were repetitions of the pattern observed during March–May. New developments occurred, different numbers were registered but the pattern remained essentially the same. It was as though a kind of fractal self-similarity was at play. The case of the state of Victoria in Australia illustrates neatly the repetitive nature of the subsequent months.

Of all the measures of state governments in Australia during April 2020, the Victorian government had the harshest shutdown. The state premier (Daniel Andrews) and his ministers underscored this with a distinctly authoritarian public tone. Yet when the Victorian government relaxed its regulations on May 13 2020, one of its first acts was to permit sizable family gatherings in spite of the clear evidence of the specific manner in which the virus was transmitted. Public pressure for family-type close social contact proved irresistible. Six weeks later, the Victorian government began to panic about the number of cases that were being passed on through extended-family networks among close-contact cultures particularly in north-western suburban outer-ring of Victoria's 5 million strong capital city, Melbourne. On July 9 the state government re-imposed broad-sweeping generic lockdown orders contrary to the pattern of virus spread which was geographically specific (north-western suburbs), socially specific (extended families, large-sized households and housing towers) and institutionally specific (nursing homes, hospitals and food processing plants). Deaths were concentrated in the over-70s and nursing home cohorts—as it proved to be in most comparable countries. The Victorian government's policy was a scatter-gun one. It attempted to "suppress" the virus as opposed to targeted mitigation focused on the diverse nature of COVID transmission and mortality.

The pattern of transmission in Victoria was the same as the international pattern. Internationally, sources of major spread (more than 20 cases of transmission) were nursing homes, labour barracks, conferences, churches, ships, food processing plants, prisons, markets, and occasionally parties and weddings.[1] Internationally, sources of mid-range spread (5–19 cases of transmission) were the same as the major spread sources with the addition of households. Transmission events related to restaurant meals (many with family and close friends), schools, hospitals, workplaces, shopping malls and sports occurred but more occasionally. At the low end of cluster spread (2–4 cases of transmission), households and family-related meals predominated alongside sporadic transmission events related to fitness classes and hospitals. Communitarian interactions were the primary transmission medium for the virus. This social pattern was reinforced by the powerful social desire for *gemeinschaft* and the consequent appetite (much of it unconscious) for all manner of close-contact social behaviour. The most robust corrective to this was the *gesellschaft*, the society of strangers interacting at a distance through contracts and other impersonal media.

The uptick of cases that occurred in Victoria in July 2020 but not across the rest of Australia reflected the pattern of geographic clustering that also was typical of the virus spread. In Victoria as in many other places this geographic clustering had a fractal character. Just as the increased spread of COVID-19 in June–August was concentrated in a single Australian state so also, within that state, the virus spread was concentrated in four local government areas in the northern and western suburbs of Melbourne. These virus cases had other characteristics familiar from across the world. The principal pattern of spread in Melbourne's northern and western suburbs was through extended families and large-sized households, and in big clusters in nursing homes and food processing plants.

The Victorian government chose not to pursue a tailored strategy focusing on (a) the known prime media of transmission (family gatherings, residential aged care and food processing factories), pathways of transmission that could be managed and mitigated, and (b) the known at-high-risk population (over-70s with comorbidities, particularly nursing home residents).

A tailored policy would have restricted extended family gatherings and installed infection control officers in all nursing homes and food processing plants in April 2020. Rather the government chose to lockdown the state not once but twice in the June–October period. After the first three-week lockdown in July the effective reproduction rate of the virus in Victoria had been reduced from 1.75 to 1.16 and below 1 on July 28 and 29.[2] A R_E of 1 is the point at which the virus spread declines. In spite of that benchmark low reproduction number having been reached, the Victorian government on the 2nd of August introduced an even more severe population-wide lockdown for a further three months. The 7-day average reproduction rate through August and September was 0.94, a recurring metrical pattern that was little changed by the lockdown. Cumulative COVID-related deaths by October 10 in Victoria amounted to 809, 2% of the 41,000 annual deaths in Victoria. Almost all of the COVID-related fatalities were aged over 70 and a very large percentage were from nursing homes.

The COVID-19 infection fatality rate (IFR) in Victoria in early October of 2020 was likely in the order of 0.2%, extrapolating from the July 2020 review of 32 serological data sets from across the world by John Ioannidis. An infection fatality rate based on serological surveys is calculated using the number of persons that anti-body (B cell) tests show to be infected. This number does not include persons who were infected but only had a T cell immune response to the virus.[3] Ioannidis found an infection fatality rate of "0.10% in locations with COVID-19 population mortality rate less than the global average (<73 deaths per million as of July 12, 2020), 0.27% in locations with 73–500 COVID-19 deaths per million, and 0.90% in locations exceeding 500 COVID-19 deaths per million".[4] On October 10 2020 the average of deaths per million across the world was 137 per million. Eighteen countries out of 215 exceeded the 500 per million upper threshold; 132 countries fell below the less than 73 per million line.[5] The 1918 Spanish flu pandemic infected a third (500 million) of the 1500 million population worldwide. 50 million of the estimated 500 million infected died, a 10% infection fatality rate and 1% of the world's population.[6] One million worldwide died from the 1957–1958 H2N2 virus pandemic (the "Asian flu"), 0.034% of the global population.[7] A million died from the 1968 H3N2 virus, 0.028% of the world's population.[8] As of October 10 2020, there had been 1,072,712 COVID-related deaths worldwide, 0.014% of the 7.8 billion global population.

Victoria was in the mid-range of the international spectrum. Its death rate at the time was 124 persons per million. The health risk to the broad public was mild. Nevertheless an aggressive shutdown of the state took place. Freedom of movement was severely curtailed as were employment and business activity. A night curfew was applied and the state parliament was furloughed. An omnipresent executive government operated through administrative direction. The primary health risk was overwhelmingly concentrated in the state's nursing homes. By the end of May 2020, 30% of COVID-related deaths in Australia had occurred in nursing homes, a moderate figure among comparable OECD countries. By October 10 the figure stood at 75% of COVID-related deaths. As of May 25 2020, nursing home deaths averaged 42% across the OECD, ranging from less than 10% in Hungary to 66% in Spain and 81% in Canada.[9] "Australia", though, is a misnomer in this context. For the change in outcomes from March–April to July–August was entirely attributable to one state, Victoria.

On October 10, there were 676 COVID-related deaths in nursing homes in Australia out of a total of 896 deaths (75%). Of the 676 aged-care mortalities, 646 (95%) had occurred in Victoria, a state with 25% of Australia's population.[10] It was possible to keep COVID-related deaths to a minimum with tailored and targeted responses including rigorous infection control in places where fatalities were concentrated, notably nursing homes.[11] In countries with comparable social systems to Victoria's, the death rate in nursing homes varied considerably: 35% (Denmark), 63% (Ireland), 64% (Belgium) and 85% (Canada).[12] Lockdowns or the severity of lockdowns had little or no correlation with these outcomes. In Sweden with mild restrictions 47% of COVID-related deaths were in nursing homes. In England and Wales with a severe lockdown of the population it was 49%.[13] Singapore had an exacting six-week lockdown with 8% only of deaths in nursing homes, off a small total per capita death rate from the virus. In contrast Japan avoided a national shutdown of its economy and society. It relied instead on its population following the government's three-C advice to avoid enclosed spaces with poor ventilation, crowded places with many people and close contact settings such as face-to-face conversations. Japan had a low per capita death rate and no excess deaths during the virus mortality peak in January through April 2020.[14] As of May 10, 60 of Japan's 624 COVID-related deaths had occurred in nursing homes, 9.6%.[15] Japan's population is 126 million.

The comparison of Victoria's (6.3 million) and Hong Kong's (7.4 million) population is instructive. Both had a second July–August wave of cases: one in winter and one in summer. Both at that point had a high percentage of deaths in nursing homes (Hong Kong 85%; Victoria 70%).[16] Yet only a tiny total of 86 deaths had occurred in Hong Kong by the end of August 2020 compared to 513 in Victoria, 6 times the Hong Kong rate. Victoria chose a strategy of sweeping shutdown. In contrast Hong Kong's restrictions on businesses, gatherings and institutions were targeted and mild while the public health outcomes were markedly better. Rather than adopting a tailored approach the Victorian government ordered a large portion of general population to stay at home under highly restrictive conditions including a curfew in order to reduce the case count among the general population whose immune system responses were robust. This was contrary to the lesson of evolution, namely that human beings over millennia have evolved a complex and still little understood immune system that is effective in fighting viruses. Even vaccines only reinforce the "memory" of a person's immune system in order to leverage the body's own defences against a virus. Most of the work of fighting viruses is done by the human body. Science to a limited degree is able to boost that. As to governments, in reality the best they can do is to (a) shelter those with weak immune systems with good advice or institutional infection control measures; and (b) implement effective infection control in places known to rapidly spread a virus.

In Victoria's case, when clusters developed, these were predictable and limited in type: nursing homes and food processing plants principally. In the case of a virus cluster, the transmission of the virus tracks not just to one or a handful of other persons as in the case of transmission via family and friends. Rather the virus reproduces itself among a significant number of persons. As of August 10 2020, 63 such virus clusters ranging in size from 10 to over 300 had been confirmed in Victoria.[17] The origin of 37% of infections in these cluster transmission chains were residential care homes, almost all of them aged care facilities. The source of 24% of cluster infections was food processing plants. Ten percent originated in public housing. Hospitals accounted for 6% and schools for 4%. Other sources were negligible. Rather than targeting the major cluster sources (aged care, food production plants and large close-contact accommodation facilities) with effective tailored infection control early on (as early as March), which was something within the capacity of government, the state opted for a late-arriving stay-at-home approach (as late as July and August) which did not stop the spread of the virus among high-risk populations. On March 27 2020 as part of a national program the state even created its own large close-contact accommodation facilities in the form of quarantine hotels for travellers returning from overseas. These facilities were badly managed and later proved to be the ultimate source of most of the subsequent confirmed virus cases in the state, spreading out from the barracks-like quarantine hotel crucible into extended family networks mostly in a geographical cluster of four northern and western suburban local government areas in Melbourne.

In Victoria during its first (March to May) lockdown, pathology cancer notifications fell by 28%. In the subsequent August to September lockdown, emergency department admissions for major fatal conditions were down 20%.[18] Self-harm admissions of children rose 33% on the previous year.[19] Vaccinations of under-five year olds dropped by 20%.[20] In July 2020 Victorian government representatives were claiming that the state's shutdown had saved "tens of thousands" of lives. Assuming an infection fatality rate of 0.25% that would have required a population twice the size of Victoria's to have been infected. Conversely on August 23 in the midst of Victoria's July–August case uptick, 585 persons were hospitalised with COVID-19, occupying 2.4% of the state's total hospital beds, far from exaggerated predictions of needs for hospital beds and resources.[21]

What would have happened to the rate of mortality if there had been no shutdown? Sweden gives us a good insight into this. Its government did not impose an official shutdown of the country though, understandably, social and economic activity did decline significantly during the virus peak. Swedish deaths per capita attributed to COVID were on the high side by global standards. The Swedes admitted that they failed to insulate their nursing homes. Even so on a year-to-year basis comparing deaths from all causes in Sweden for the months July–June for the years 2015–16 through 2019–20, the death tally of the last year—the COVID year—was 105% (2015–2016), 102% (2016–2017), 103% (2017–2018), and 106% (2018–2019) of the preceding years.[22] That is, in Sweden the excess death rate spike in March–April 2020 attributable to COVID did not translate into a markedly higher annual incidence of deaths compared to recent prior years. Deaths per year commonly approach one percent of a population. In England and Wales in 2016–2017, it was 0.90% and in 2017–18, 0.91%. In 2019–2020 all deaths totalled 0.98%.[23] Did the modest addition of 0.08% deaths in 2019–2020 over 2016–2017 justify the United Kingdom shutting down its economy and society for multiple weeks?

In mid-July 2020, four months after shutdown policies were implemented in the United Kingdom, the British government produced an actuarial report on projected mortality and morbidity in coming decades from the UK lockdown.[24] The report paints a picture of indirect deaths and loss of life-span that far outweighs the number of COVID-related deaths. In the UK between March 21 and May 1 2020 there were 32,000 COVID-related deaths, of which 25,000 were "excess deaths" which would not have occurred otherwise within a year. Compare this to the public policy related non-COVID deaths: it is estimated in the same period that (a) changes to emergency hospital care accounted for 6000 excess deaths, (b) changes to primary and preventive care in nursing homes accounted for 10,000 excess deaths, and (c) postponing or cancelling elective care was responsible for 12,500 excess deaths. Changes to community and primary care accounted for an additional 1400 excess deaths. There were some positives from the UK's lockdown including fewer deaths from road accidents and childhood infections, accounting for 3000 less deaths. In short as many excess deaths occurred in April 2020 in the United Kingdom because of COVID public policy as occurred because of COVID.

What about the future? Mortality as a result of recession is pro-cyclical (the immediate effect of a recession is to reduce death rates) resulting in an expected 4500 fewer excess deaths within the year following the UK's 2020 lockdown. But within 2–5 years the negative health effects of recession kick in, with a resulting 18,000 excess deaths anticipated. And in the longer term, more than five years into the future? The UK's official actuaries predict a further 15,000 excess deaths, the equivalent of 438,000 quality-adjusted life years (QALYs) lost.[25] The long-term excess deaths result from the elevated mortality rate of young adults caught in a severe recession. As of August 30 2020, Britain had 41,498 COVID-related deaths. By the count of its own actuary's office, Britain's COVID public policy will be responsible for 55,400 excess deaths in the short term due to shutdown [March and April only were included in the count] and in the medium and longer term due to the effects of lockdown-induced recession on mortality. In the end, the cure for the disease will prove worse than the disease itself.

NOTES

1. Leclerc et al. (2020)
2. Bennett (2020) and Saul (2020).
3. Gallais (2020). This study examined immune responses against COVID in 7 families including nine index patients with mild cases of COVID-19 and eight contacts. Six of the eight contacts reported COVID symptoms 1–7 days after the index patients. The six contacts all tested seronegative (no antibodies) but positive for COVID-specific T cell immune responses.

4. Ioannidis, July 14, 2020, p. 2.
5. Worldometer, Coronavirus, 11 August 2020.
6. US Centres for Disease Control, 1918 Pandemic (H1N1 virus).
7. US Centres for Disease Control, 1957–1958 Pandemic (H2N2 virus).
8. US Centres for Disease Control, 1968 Pandemic (H3N2 virus).
9. Canadian Institute for Health Information, June 2020.
10. Commonwealth Department of Health data, 8 August 2020.
11. Gilbert (2020) provides an Australian study of an early (March) example of failed infection prevention and control at the Dorothy Henderson Lodge nursing home in New South Wales.
12. Comas-Herrera et al. (2020, Table 1).
13. UK Office of National Statistics, Deaths involving COVID-19 in the care sector, England and Wales: deaths occurring up to 12 June 2020 and registered up to 20 June 2020 (provisional).
14. Japan Ministry of Health, Labour and Welfare.
15. Lies (2020).
16. Hong (2020).
17. Victorian Department of Health data aggregated by www.covid19data.com.au
18. Kehoe (2020).
19. Clayton (2020).
20. Royal Children's Hospital survey of 2000 parents.
21. Hospital bed count, Australian Institute of Health and Welfare, Hospital resources 2017–18: Australian hospital statistics.
22. SCB, Number of deaths reported to Statistics Sweden, per day for 2015–20,201 (entire country), Table 1.
23. UK Office of National Statistics, Deaths registered weekly in England and Wales, provisional.
24. Department of Health and Social Care, 15 July 2020.
25. On this measure 1 life year is one year of life lived in perfect health; a quality-adjusted year depends on a person's state of health. A person in bad health might be 0.3; a dead person is 0.

References

Bennett, C. (2020, August 6). Figure: Reproductive factor of the virus. When will Victoria's daily coronavirus numbers start to come down? *The Age*.

Canadian Institute for Health Information. (2020, June). Pandemic Experience in the Long-Term Care Sector: How Does Canada Compare With Other Countries? *CIHI Snapshot*.

Clayton, R. (2020, August 8). Statistics show increase in children presenting to hospitals after self-harming. *ABC News*.

Comas-Herrera, A. et al. (2020, June 26). *Mortality associated with COVID-19 outbreaks in care homes: early international evidence.* International Long Term Care Policy Network.

Department of Health and Social Care, Office for National Statistics, Government Actuary's Department and Home Office. (2020, July 15). *Direct and Indirect Impacts of COVID-19 on Excess Deaths and Morbidity.* UK Government.

Ioannidis, J. (2020, July 14). The infection fatality rate of COVID-19 inferred from seroprevalence data. *medRxiv* preprint. https://doi.org/10.1101/2020.05.13.20101253

Gallais, F. (2020, June 22). Intrafamilial Exposure to SARS-CoV-2 Induces Cellular Immune Response without Seroconversion. *medRxiv* preprint. https://doi.org/10.1101/2020.06.21.20132449

Gilbert, G. (2020, July 17). COVID-19 in a Sydney nursing home: a case study and lessons learnt. *The Medical Journal of Australia* preprint. https://www.mja.com.au/system/files/2020-07/Gilbert%20mja20.01238%20-%2017%20July%202020.pdf

Hong, J. (2020, August 10). Nursing Home Outbreaks Lift Death Rates in Hong Kong, Australia. *Bloomberg.*

Keheo, J. (2020, August 12). More cancer deaths from COVID-19 lockdown. *Australian Financial Review.*

Leclerc, Q. J. et al. (2020). What settings have been linked to SARS-CoV-2 transmission clusters? *Wellcome Open Research* 5:83.

Lies, E. (2020, May 12) In Japan's elder-care homes, coronavirus tests limits of overstretched staff. *Reuters.*

Saul, A. (2020, 4 August) Victoria's response to a resurgence of COVID-19 has averted 9,000–37,000 cases in July 2020. *Medical Journal of Australia* preprint.

Index[1]

A
Abstemiousness, 93
Acquaintances, 22, 60, 68, 102
Adaptation, 3, 51
Air quality, 15
Analogies, 54
Antibodies, 3, 33n12, 61
Antinomy of freedom, 96
Anxieties, 47–49, 54, 69, 72, 76, 77, 88, 89, 100–102
Apocalypse, 56, 87
Apocalyptic, 54, 55, 78n3, 87, 88, 94
Asceticism, 93
Ascetic priests, 93
Asymptomatic, 32n3, 48, 54
Attack rate, 20, 34n23, 46, 79n20, 97
Australia, 4, 46, 48, 62, 70, 75, 78n11, 80n27, 104n2
Authentic, 101
Authoritarian, 99
Autonomous solidarity, 31

B
Balance, 73, 91
Balancing of competing considerations, 71
Bans on gatherings, 45, 49
Basic reproduction number, 2, 52
Beliefs, 87, 97–104
Bell curve, 12, 50, 51, 56, 64, 86
Border closures, 45
Broadcasters, 86
Bureaucratic state, 92

C
Calm, 88, 101
Canada, 4, 7, 22, 70
Case fatality rate, 11
Catastrophic, 86, 88
Catastrophism, 87–88
Causality, 4, 31, 50, 64
Cause, 21, 72, 79n25, 96, 97, 100, 102

---

[1] Note: Page numbers followed by 'n' refer to notes.

Certainty, 92, 97
Change, 78n3, 103
Charisma, 99
Charismatic, 21, 99, 103
Children, 21, 34n23, 46, 47, 60, 77n2, 93, 96, 101
China, 19–21, 31, 46, 52, 63, 69, 70, 78n3, 78n13, 79n20, 93, 99
Chronic underlying health conditions, 60
Civic, 29, 49
Clichés, 87
Climate, 15, 31
Close contacts, 20, 21, 46, 68
Closed commercial state, 93
Closeness, 62, 67, 68, 101
Clusters, 19, 21, 34n24, 60, 79n20, 89
Collective hysteria, 86
Communicable, 77, 86, 88
Communism, 92
Community contacts, 20
Community immunity, 2, 3, 11, 44, 67, 77n1
Co-morbidities, 3, 72
Competing goods, 71, 73, 91
Conspiracy theories, 97
Contingencies, 52, 97
Control, 3, 21, 49, 62, 63, 67, 75, 89, 95, 100, 103
Coronavirus, 60, 78n3
Costs and benefits, 75, 90
COVID-19, 2–4, 7, 11, 15, 21, 22, 29, 31, 32n4, 32n6, 32n7, 33n13, 34n15, 34n18, 34n19, 44, 46, 47, 49–51, 56, 59, 60, 67, 72, 73, 78n15, 79n20, 79n25, 80n26, 86, 87, 90, 94, 103
Crowded, 19, 21, 22, 31, 34n18, 49
Crowds, 19
Cruise, 21, 34n24, 67, 78n15
Customs, 98

D
Danish, 75
Death, 3, 4, 7, 11, 12, 15, 22, 29, 31, 32n4, 32n7, 33n12, 34n19, 47, 48, 50, 51, 56, 59, 62, 64, 72, 73, 75, 78n6, 78n13, 79n22, 80n26, 80n27, 85, 86, 90, 91, 98–100, 102–103
Depression, 69, 88
Differentiated, 61, 94
Distance, 11, 22, 29, 39, 45, 49, 62, 68, 97, 101, 102
Distancing, 11, 22, 39, 44, 45, 50, 51, 63, 64, 68, 69, 73, 75, 96, 102
Durkheim, Emile, 94

E
Economic and social costs, 69
Economic stimulus, 70
Effective reproduction number, 2, 51, 64, 75, 86
Emergency state, 92, 94–95
Empirical, 54, 55, 60, 90, 97
Empirical evidence, 54, 97
Enclosed spaces, 19, 34n18, 49
End-of-the world, 88
Entertainment, 19, 61, 105n2
Epidemiarchy, 99
Epidemiologists, 2, 50, 68, 105n3
Equilibrium, 91
Estonia, 62, 78n11
Exceptional authority, 94
Excess deaths, 7, 32n7, 72, 73
Exogenous impacts, 93
Exogenous shocks, 1
Explanations, 15, 97, 99
Expressivism, 96, 102

F
Family, 19–21, 29, 34n24, 49, 60
Family members, 19, 20
Fantasies, 102

Farr, William, 12, 50
Fear of death, 100
Fears, 72, 73, 102
Ferguson, Professor Neil, 56
Ferguson report, 56–63
Finitude, 100
Flatten the curve, 87
Fractal, 22, 31, 61
France, 4, 22, 33n11, 34n24, 61, 70
Freedom, 93, 96
Freedom of movement, 93, 99
Free will, 103
Friends, 20, 22, 29, 46, 60, 68
Futurism, 89

G
Global Financial Crisis of 2008, 88
God, 87, 102–103
Good judgment, 71
Government, 3, 44, 47–51, 55, 56, 60–63, 67–69, 71, 73, 86, 92, 94, 95, 99, 104, 104n2

H
Habits of a society, 98
Hairdressing, 15
Hall, Edward T., 22
Hawkishness, 54
Headlines, 87
Health care, 20
Herd immunity, 2, 11, 61, 67
Hero, 98, 99
Heroism, 98–99
High-contact culture, 22
High-touch society, 49
Home, 4, 19, 29, 39, 45, 47, 49, 62, 63, 68, 73, 94–96, 98
Hospital, 4, 19, 34n18, 45, 47–52, 54, 63, 68, 73, 78n4, 78n6, 80n26, 91, 98
Hospital beds, 51, 54

Household members, 20
Households, 20, 21, 34n23, 63, 64, 68, 69, 79n20, 94
Hubei, 19, 34n23, 63, 78n13
Humility, 59
Hungary, 4
Hunt, Jeremy, 48

I
ICU, 98
Ideologies, 95
Immune, 2, 3, 33n9, 54, 67, 93
Immunity, 2, 3, 7, 11, 33n8, 44, 67
Imperial College, 32n7, 56, 62–64, 67–69, 75
Infantilize, 96
Infection fatality rate, 11, 12, 15, 63
Influenza, 2, 11, 12, 15, 52, 77n3, 85
Institutional priorities, 47
Institutions, 98
Instructions, 95, 103
Intervention, 51, 63, 67, 69, 99, 100
Intimate diffidence, 31
Italy, 15, 22, 29, 32n4, 62, 70, 78n11

J
Japan, 21, 50, 62, 70, 78n11
Japan's Ministry of Health, 50
Judgment, 71, 91

L
Law, 60
Liberalism, 92
Limits, 3, 62, 95, 100
Lockdowns, 2, 29, 49, 50, 52, 61, 62, 69, 70, 75, 79n25, 92–94, 96, 104
Loss of life-span years, 73
Lum, Professor Terry, 48

M

Macro-scale, 104
Macro-social, 21, 31
Mass events, 89, 90, 95, 97, 99
Mass social events, 97, 99
Meaning, 86, 100, 103
Mechanical solidarity, 94
Media, 86, 87, 89
Metrical realist, 90, 91
Michigan, 48
Micro-social, 21, 31, 101
Middle way, 71
Mid-range, 49, 56
Mitigation, 63, 68, 95, 96
Modellers, 54, 95
Modelling, 48, 51, 54, 59, 89, 95
Models, 3, 54
Moralising, 92
Moralism, 91–92
Mortality, 2–15, 29, 72, 73, 79n25, 97, 100
Multi-generational households, 15
Multiple causal factors, 55
Myth, 99, 101

N

Newspapers, 86
New York, 4, 31, 32n4, 33n11, 35n31, 47, 48, 73
Norway, 4, 29, 70, 75
Novel event, 54
Nursing homes, 4, 21, 29, 46–48, 69, 96

O

Objectivism, 102
Objectivity, 101
Observation, 22, 49, 54, 88, 89, 97
Observation of reality, 88
Oracles, 89

Organic solidarity, 94
Organizations, 98
Outdoors, 19

P

Pandemics, 56, 86, 95, 97
Paradox, 29
Pathogen, 3, 11, 71, 86, 96
Patterns, 11, 12, 21, 31, 34n25, 47, 51, 54, 56, 60, 62, 73, 79n18, 89, 90, 97, 101
Personal space, 22, 29, 31, 32
Pessimism, 88–89
Physical contact, 15, 20, 31, 46, 67–69
Physical interaction, 44
Planners, 54, 95
Planning state, 92
Pluralism, 91
Population density, 31, 61
Predictions of disaster, 88
Procedural, 54, 98
Proportionality, 49–56, 71, 96
Providence, 103
Proxemics, 22, 101
Proximity, 15, 20, 21, 29, 47, 62, 101
Prudence, 71, 91
Prudent, 49, 69, 73, 102
Prudential, 71, 78n3, 88
Pseudo church, 103
Public health, 45–48, 56, 60, 72, 77n1, 86, 94, 105n2
Public opinion, 85–87, 91, 92, 100
Publics, 86, 97, 101, 103, 104

Q

Quantum, 91
Quarantining, 45, 50, 54
Queensland, 46

R

Rationalism, 90–91
Realism, 89–90
Reality, 59, 80n27, 87, 89, 95, 99
Recession, 73
Reclusive conviviality, 31
Redemptive politics, 103
Regions, 4, 7, 11, 12, 15, 22, 29, 31, 33n13, 50, 60, 72
Regulations, 60
Relatives, 19, 20, 46, 49, 60, 68
Religion, 103
Restaurants, 15, 19
Restrictions, 2, 21, 45, 49, 63, 75, 105n2
Rhetoric of emergency, 49
Romanticism, 93, 101
Rules, 98
Rules of institutions, 98

S

School closures, 45
Seasonal influenza, 2
Secular redemption, 103
Self-certitude, 92, 97
Self-organizing, 54
Self-responsibility, 96
Shock events, 89, 95
Shutdown, 19, 39, 54, 59, 63, 69, 75, 80n27, 86, 94, 99
Shuttered society, 93
Singapore, 4, 21, 34n24, 48
Single households, 15
Smoking, 15
Sociable autonomy, 31
Social causation, 55
Social contagion, 55
Social distancing, 45–46
Socialism, 92, 94, 96
Socially-connected individuals, 19
Social media, 86, 87, 89
South Korea, 2, 21, 34n24, 62, 70, 78n11
Spain, 4, 29, 33n11, 61, 62, 70, 78n11
Stoicism, 103–104
Strangers, 19, 22, 68, 69, 100–102
Suffering, 103
Supermarkets, 15, 19
Suppression, 59, 63, 64, 89
Suppression strategies, 59
Surfaces, 19, 45

T

Taiwan, 15, 20, 62, 78n11
Targeted, 46, 49, 50, 60, 96
Temperature, 15, 31, 35n32
Testing, 45, 47, 61, 78n3, 86
Totalitarian, 93, 94
Touch, 19, 21, 22, 49, 101
Tracing, 21, 45, 50, 69
Transmission, 3, 15, 19–21, 31, 32n3, 34n18, 34n23, 46, 49, 51, 63, 68, 69, 79n18, 79n20, 98, 101
Transport, 19, 68, 104n2

U

Uncertainty, 71, 92, 102
Underlying conditions, 4, 47
Unemployment, 70, 73, 79n25
Uniform, 60
Uninhibited, 3, 100
Unintended consequences, 69–77, 95
United Kingdom, 47, 50, 59, 62, 72, 78n11, 103
United States, 4, 7, 12, 22, 48, 49, 70, 72, 79n25
Urban density, 31, 61

V

Vaccine, 3, 7, 11, 44
Variation in exposure, 67, 68
Variation in individual
    susceptibility, 67, 68
Virus, 2–4, 7, 11, 12, 15, 19–21, 29,
    31, 33n8, 33n13, 34n22, 39,
    44–47, 49, 50, 52, 54, 59–63,
    67–69, 72, 73, 75, 76, 78n3,
    78n6, 78n15, 78n16, 79n20,
    80n26, 80n27, 85, 86, 90, 95,
    96, 98, 100, 101, 104n1, 104n2

W

WHO, *see* World Health Organization
Will to believe,
    97, 99
Workplace, 19, 64, 68
World Health Organization (WHO),
    46, 68, 77n3,
    78n4, 78n6,
    79n20, 105n3
Wuhan, 2, 19, 32n4,
    33n11, 34n18, 47, 63,
    77n2, 78n4

The manufacturer's authorised representative in the EU is Springer Nature Customer Service Centre GmbH, Europaplatz 3, 69115 Heidelberg, Germany. If you have any concerns regarding our products, please contact ProductSafety@springernature.com

Printed and bound by CPI Group (UK) Ltd, Croydon, CR0 4YY
25/03/2026
02078197-0002